Hospital Administrator's Desk Book

Hospital Administrator's Desk Book

Robert C. Benjamin
Rudolph C. Kemppainen

Prentice-Hall, Inc.   •   Englewood Cliffs, New Jersey

Prentice-Hall International, Inc., *London*
Prentice-Hall of Australia, Pty, Ltd., *Sydney*
Prentice-Hall Canada, Inc., *Toronto*
Prentice-Hall of India Private, Ltd., *New Delhi*
Prentice-Hall of Japan, Inc., *Tokyo*
Prentice-Hall of Southeast Asia Pte, Ltd., *Singapore*
Whitehall Books, Ltd., Wellington, *New Zealand*
Editora Prentice-Hall do Brazil Ltda., *Rio de Janeiro*

© 1983 *by*

PRENTICE-HALL, INC.
Englewood Cliffs, N.J.

"This publication is designed to provide accurate and authoritative
information in regard to the subject matter covered. It is sold with
the understanding that the publisher is not engaged in rendering
legal, accounting, or other professional service. If legal advice or
other expert assistance is required, the services of a competent
professional person should be sought."
—*From the Declaration of Principles jointly adopted by a
Committee of the American Bar Association and a Committee
of Publishers and Associations.*

Library of Congress Cataloging in Publication Data
Benjamin, Robert C.
   Hospital administrator's desk book.

   Includes index.
   1. Hospitals—Administration. I. Kemppainen,
Rudolph C., 1952-   • II. Title.
RA971.B374 1983   362.1'1068   82-14980
ISBN 0-13-394890-0

Printed in the United States of America

THE AUTHORS

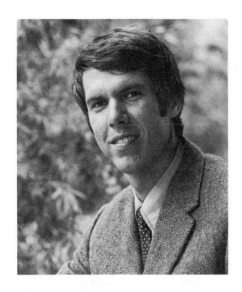

Robert C. Benjamin

Robert C. Benjamin of Casa Grande, Arizona, has an impressive background of successful hospital administration. After receiving his Bachelor of Business Administration degree from Tulane University of Louisiana in 1967, he served a tour of duty with the U.S. Army Medical Service Corps, with assignments in the Republic of South Vietnam and Munich, Germany. After completing his military tour, he furthered his education with a Master of Business Administration degree from Michigan State University in 1971 and Post Master's Certificate in Health Care administration from George Washington University of Washington, D.C., in 1973.

His unique brand of administrative vision has been felt in such diverse places as Lancaster General Hospital of Pennsylvania, Portage View Hospital of Hancock, Michigan, the Clinica Santa Maria of Santiago, Chile, to his current position as administrator of Hoemako Hospital of Casa Grande, Arizona.

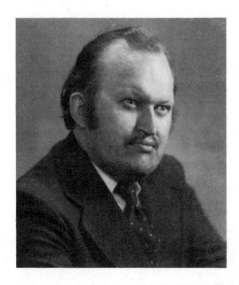

Rudolph C. Kemppainen

Rudolph C. Kemppainen of Chassell, Michigan, has an extensive background in business-product consulting, marketing, and motivational technique development. From this background, he conducted extensive research into effective health care delivery systems.

His writing background includes articles on sales and motivation psychology techniques. He also has one previous book co-authorship to his credit: *Building The $100,000 Dental Practice,* (C) 1981 by Prentice-Hall, Inc.

What This Desk Book Will Do
For You and Your Hospital

AS A HOSPITAL ADMINISTRATOR, you're on the "hot seat." Presented with problems and challenges of increasing complexity, you are faced with decisions that can have a profound effect on the community you serve.

As the head of a major financial force within the community, you are faced with the dilemma of maintaining a high quality of health service while holding the line on the cost. Ever-increasing pressure is being brought from consumer and government agencies to decrease the inflation rate of hospital care.

To achieve this goal, your task is to mold numerous departments, with differing problems and viewpoints, into a smooth-running machine. The job can be a source of great personal and professional satisfaction; or it can be as nerve-wracking as tip-toeing through a mine field. Much depends on the approach you take.

Without realizing it, many administrators become so attached to facts and figures that they lose sight of the human aspects of their position. By placing a disproportionate emphasis on the final result, as opposed to how it is achieved, a human relations "nightmare" can be created.

As a direct result, optimum hospital operation is sacrificed. In order to make this book an effective working tool for you, our goal is to capture the heartbeat of a well-managed hospital, offering a yardstick by which you can make realistic judgments on the effectiveness of your operations.

We will explore the functioning of the "vital organs" of a hospital, the various departmental services. Examining the situation from both administrative and departmental viewpoints, we will help you to pinpoint the most common problems you'll face and offer possible solutions.

Here is a partial list of answers to everyday challenges this book will address:

- EFFECTIVE COMMUNICATIONS TECHNIQUES FOR THE ADMINISTRATOR.
- PROVEN METHODS FOR GETTING ALONG WITH THE MEDICAL STAFF.
- HOW TO FORMULATE AN EFFECTIVE BUDGET.
- THE FOUR PHASES OF EFFECTIVE PERSONNEL MANAGEMENT.
- HOW TO EFFECTIVELY HANDLE COLLECTIVE BARGAINING AND UNION PROBLEMS.
- PROS AND CONS OF GROUP BUYING.
- COMPUTER UTILIZATION IN INVENTORY CONTROL.
- HOW TO USE MEDICAL RECORDS TO EVALUATE HEALTH CARE EFFECTIVENESS.

- COST-CUTTING THROUGH EFFECTIVE PREVENTIVE MAINTENANCE.
- HOW TO INCREASE THE EFFICIENCY OF THE HOUSEKEEPING DEPARTMENT.
- NEW TECHNIQUES FOR THE HOSPITAL LAUNDRY.
- HOW TO PLAN AN EFFECTIVE HOSPITAL SECURITY SYSTEM.
- EFFECTIVE ADMINISTRATIVE AIDS FOR THE NURSING SERVICE.
- EFFECTIVE COST ACCOUNTING PROCEDURES FOR LAB SERVICES.
- INCREASING THE SAFETY AND EFFICIENCY OF THE RADIOLOGY DEPARTMENT.
- COST RATIOS OF IN-HOUSE VS. CONSULTING SERVICE PHARMACY.
- HOW TO ELIMINATE FRICTION BETWEEN DIETARY AND NURSING SERVICES.
- HOW TO EFFECTIVELY COORDINATE PHYSICAL MEDICINE AND REHABILITATION SERVICES.
- HOW TO ORGANIZE EFFECTIVE IN-SERVICE TRAINING FOR EMPLOYEES.
- HOW TO EXPAND AVAILABLE REVENUE WITH CREATIVE UTILIZATION PRACTICES.
- HOW TO RECRUIT PHYSICIANS AND OTHER SPECIALIZED PERSONNEL.
- HOW TO ESTABLISH EFFECTIVE COMMUNICATIONS WITH THE SURROUNDING COMMUNITY.
- HOW TO QUALIFY FOR, AND DELIVER, FEDERAL AND OTHER GOVERNMENT FUNDING.
- FUTURE TRENDS FOR HOSPITALS.

A detailed re-examination of our health care delivery system is required as a prerequisite to responding to public needs. Your obligation is to review your present operating procedures to spot any deficiencies.

This book will help you in this task. In the upcoming pages, we will present the diagnostic tools and offer curative steps as required. Using examples that have worked for other hospitals, we will show how potentially bad situations can be turned around.

With knowledge, determination, and some innovative thinking, you and your hospital can join the vanguard of top hospitals as models of managerial excellence.

An action program for bottom line results is at your fingertips.

Robert C. Benjamin
Rudolph C. Kemppainen

(For further information on specific aspects of hospital management, the reader is referred to the Prentice-Hall *Hospital Cost Management Loose-Leaf Service,* by John G. Steinle.)

CONTENTS

Chapter 1

**HOW TO AVOID THE NUMBER ONE PITFALL OF
HOSPITAL ADMINISTRATION** 21

Answers to breakdowns in communications — the number one
problem — "two way" links in the process — use of money as
an incentive — "selling" administrative ideas effectively —
setting realistic goals — getting people mobilized

Chapter 2

**TESTED SUCCESSFUL ORGANIZATION PRINCIPLES FOR
YOUR HOSPITAL** 27

Covers the basic "skeletal structure" of sound hospital
management. Includes: minimum departmental requirements
— dietary department — medical records department — the
pharmacy — laboratories — radiology — emergency service —
the medical library — optional services — outpatient
department — rehabilitation department — medical social
services department. The following are covered in a
non-specific manner: navigating storms in organizational
structure — insurance programs; public and private —
prepayment plans — future challenges — qualifications of the
administrator

Chapter 3

THE MEDICAL CORE OF HOSPITAL MANAGEMENT 40

**Part 1—How to Organize an Effective and Efficient Hospital
Staff** 41

Six essential duties of the medical staff structure — general
staff member responsibility — staff "politics" and medical
standards — internal medical staff organization — Chief of

The Medical Core of Hospital Management *(cont.)*

> Staff — the Executive Committee — the Joint Conference
> Committee — the Credentials Committee — the Medical
> Records Committee — summary of 26 common reports — the
> Tissue Committee — the Medical Audit Committee — the
> Infection Committee — policy structure for effective infection
> control — the Utilization Committee and its responsibilities

**Part 2—How to Maintain an Effective Working Relationship with
Your Medical Staff** 51

> Active administrative involvement — strengthening ties
> between hospital and medical staff — shared billing systems —
> cooperative purchasing agreements — special legal advisory —
> Benefits: the key to physician loyalty

Chapter 4

HOW TO AVOID AN ADVERSARY RELATIONSHIP WITH
YOUR BOARD OF TRUSTEES 56

> Composition of hospital boards — continuity vs. "new
> blood" — continuing education of board members — basic
> organizational framework from the hospital board
> viewpoint — the Executive Committee — the Joint
> Conference Committee — the Professional Committee — the
> Finance Committee — mutual trust as a key element —
> formal administrative presentations to the board — dangers of
> "conflict of interest" — final thoughts on the relationship
> between administration and the hospital board

Chapter 5

THE KEY SERVICE FOR HOSPITAL SOLVENCY 67

> Critical functions of the Business Office — primary
> functions — qualifications at the helm — solid working
> relationship between administrator and controller — the
> admitting office — elements of effective admission policy —
> Key $ and Timesaver — the Accounting Department — use of
> effective paper work formats — "semi-computer" technology
> — combining ideas for greater payoffs — the Paper Traffic
> Center — payroll function — the third-party payment process
> — checklist for "direct line" computer use — special problems
> of credit and collection — some peripheral functions of the
> Business Office

Chapter 6

HOW TO PLAN AN EFFECTIVE HOSPITAL BUDGET 82

Departmental budgets as a first step — specific elements of a departmental budget, including: staff salaries — supply costs — projected replacement of equipment — energy expenditures — contingency funds. Developing a total hospital budget — hospital resurrection through the Capital Outlay budget — first signs of crisis — wrapping up the budget process

Chapter 7

EFFECTIVE HUMAN RESOURCES MANAGEMENT TECHNIQUES 92

Preliminary ideas of effective personnel office techniques — qualifications of the Personnel Director — formal hospital personnel policies: an overview — conditions of employment — promotions and transfers — employment termination — merit rating system — employee services — general labor policies — health and hospitalization — hospital holidays — working hours — sick leave benefits and restrictions — rules for leave of absence — safety conditions — employee training — vacations — salary and wage policies — job analysis and description — miscellaneous policy considerations — hospital policy and employee morale — administrative role in implementation

Chapter 8

PROFITABLE PURCHASING AND MATERIALS MANAGEMENT PRACTICES 104

Defining purchasing department responsibility in general terms — dealing in specifics — purchase centralization — modified practice for specialized purchases — board-granted authority — vendor selection — quantity decisions — cost factors — the quality monitoring function — basic supply management regulations — use of computers in purchasing practice — computer inventory control — use of effective group buying practices — the legal obligations of group buying — the role of the administrator in purchase management

Chapter 9

EFFECTIVE MEDICAL RECORDS MANAGEMENT: KEY ELEMENT OF HOSPITAL EFFICIENCY

EFFECTIVE MEDICAL RECORDS MANAGEMENT: KEY ELEMENT OF HOSPITAL EFFICIENCY **114**

> Duties of the modern Medical Records Administrator — general overview of departmental objectives — needs in patient care — medical and related education's use of records — records for research use — legal considerations — the use of medical records in the administrative function — alternate techniques for better medical records efficiency — two levels of problem-solving

Chapter 10

ESSENTIAL STEPS FOR ORGANIZING EFFECTIVE ENGINEERING AND MAINTENANCE SERVICES **124**

> Departmental organization and staffing — efficient use of recorded information — the controversy over the use of an internal department vs. contracted services — benefits of an in-house maintenance program — the role of maintenance in energy conservation — maintenance department control mechanisms from an administrative perspective — analyzing departmental effectiveness

Chapter 11

THE HIDDEN LINKS TO HOSPITAL EFFICIENCY **131**

Part 1—How to Develop an Efficient Housekeeping Department **132**

> Details of housekeeping staff structure — developing effective staff training programs — the team concept for greater efficiency — housekeeping's fire and safety duties — benefits from innovative approaches

Part 2—Management Guide to Laundry and Linen **137**

> Covers organization and staffing requirements — the use of contract laundry services — consolidation of laundry services as an economy move — proper location of laundry facilities — internal structural features — how to improve laundry production

Part 3—Organizing an Effective Hospital Security Service **142**

> Criteria for implementing a hospital security service — the use of hospital-sponsored security — how to organize a security

The Hidden Links to Hospital Efficiency *(cont.)*

department — use of security in fire safety planning — special problems of handling convicts — shared facility with police agencies concept — the relationship between hospital staff and police personnel — use of video cameras in security work — granting special "arrest powers" to security staffers

Chapter 12

TEAM CONCEPTS AND PROCEDURES FOR THE NURSING STAFF **150**

Nursing staff development criteria — role of the Nursing Director — unit authority substructure — efficient centralized location of nursing station facilities — handling the medical supply connection — proper staffing levels for efficiency — innovative nurse retention programs — staff-initiated nursing programs — the nurse internship program — nursing procedural manuals — the special non-technical role of the nurse in health care delivery

Chapter 13

HOW TO MAINTAIN AND ENHANCE EFFICIENCY IN LABORATORY SERVICES **161**

Pinpoints differences between "clinical lab" and "clinical pathology" — departmental organization requirements — variable layout planning — administrative area office requirements — requirements of the technical area — auxiliary area needs — methods for expanded use — the role of public insurance in laboratory management — requirements for forms and records — special challenges in acquiring autopsy approval — use of computers in effective laboratory management

Chapter 14

THE KEY ELEMENTS FOR EFFECTIVE AND EFFICIENT RADIOLOGY SERVICES **171**

Covers departmental organization and staffing — proper construction of departmental facilities — the waiting room — radiologist's office — radiographic room's detailed requirements —

The Key Elements for Effective and Efficient Radiology Services *(cont.)*

> proper construction of the darkroom facility —
> computer advancement of radiology processes — standard
> departmental policies — the role of safety efforts in liability
> insurance costs — new trends for the future

Chapter 15

ORGANIZING AN EFFICIENT HOSPITAL PHARMACY 179

> The pharmacy's role in the hospital's clinical mission —
> criteria for choice between an in-house service and a
> consulting service pharmacy operation — the proper
> pharmacy department authority structure — the role of the
> chief pharmacist — requirements of pharmacy facilities —
> special security problems affecting pharmacy operation —
> four ideas to solve security problems — criteria for additional
> pharmacy staffing — the battle over "generics" —
> departmental paper work requirements — the administrative
> role in pharmacy efficiency

Chapter 16

**DYNAMIC MANAGEMENT CONCEPTS FOR DIETARY
SERVICES** 189

> Covers the primary function of the dietician — use of a Food
> Service Manager — proper staffing levels for a dietary
> department — use of contracted services — comparison of
> centralized and decentralized dietary services — handling the
> feeding of hospital employees — new sources of dietary
> department revenue — the question of utilizing frozen
> foods — the administrator's role in department operations

Chapter 17

**THE TWO PHASES OF RESPONSIBLE SOCIAL SERVICES
PLANNING** 200

> Targets the dual challenges to social services departments —
> proper organization of the social services department —
> relationship between medical staff and social services —
> connections with outside agencies — special challenges in cases

The Two Phases of Responsible Social Services Planning *(cont.)*

of rape — social services' responsibilities with terminally ill patients and their relatives — measuring departmental results — detailed explanation of difference between hospital and community social services workers — special thoughts on the administrator's role

Chapter 18

COORDINATED PLANNING STEPS FOR THE
MULTI-FACETED REHABILITATION SERVICES 211

Overview of nine possible departments; dealing in specifics — the medical section — the physical therapy department — occupational therapy department — psychological services — the role of social services in rehabilitation — vocational counseling — pre-vocational evaluation — rehabilitation nursing — coordinating the team effort — the regional rehabilitation center concept — using scheduling as an efficiency tool — alternate cost-savings techniques — the administrator's role

Chapter 19

KEY ELEMENTS OF INNOVATIVE HOSPITAL
EDUCATIONAL PROGRAMMING 222

Overview of hospital educational functions — developing in-service training programs — education's role in the hospital's budget — using VCR systems as a training aid — "satellite" training programs — expanding existing educational programs — community educational programming — utilizing low cost educational resource programs — the administrator's role in progressive hospital educational programming

Chapter 20

SUCCESSFUL UTILIZATION PLANS FOR VOLUNTEER
SERVICES 232

Covers special financial role of volunteers in hospital management — the hospital's Guild activities — effective

Successful Utilization Plans for Volunteer Services *(cont.)*

> volunteer recruitment techniques — special motivation keys for volunteer performance — proper coordination of volunteer activity with staff function — role of the chaplaincy program — proper chaplaincy procedures — special thoughts on volunteer non-financial contributions to hospital's quality of life

Chapter 21

EXPAND YOUR HOSPITAL'S REVENUE BASE WITH INNOVATIVE TECHNIQUES 239

> New ideas for hospital income potential — dropping departmental stereotypes — selling peripheral services to the community — special ideas for the business office — fund raising through the hospital communications system — expanded income sources through hospital lab facilities — other assorted ideas — two special questions for judging hospital revenue potential

Chapter 22

PHYSICIAN RECRUITMENT: UNVEILING THE SECRETS OF SUCCESS 245

> Factors which affect a physician's choice of hospitals — physician's daily activities — community involvement in the recruitment process — facility modification for specialized requirements — using financial inducements in the process — the unique challenges of attracting medical and surgical specialists — eliminating possible resistance from current staffers to specialty recruitment — future changes in recruiting strategy due to job market conditions — the rewards of recruiting success.

INDEX 255

Hospital Administrator's
Desk Book

How to avoid the number one pitfall of hospital administration

As WE DISCUSSED BRIEFLY IN THE INTRODUCTION to this book, hospital administrators are in a period of change—from which spring great opportunities. The greatest medical and technological advancements in the history of hospital care have happened in the past two decades. The foreseeable future shows an acceleration of these advances.

With these changes, the benefits of hospital care have been expanded far beyond the dreams of even the most progressive analysts of three and four decades ago. But these advancements have had a price.

Intricate sociological questions have been raised by the fact that some members of our society may not be able to afford the health care they might need. This is the dilemma that has forced the issue of health care and its costs into the national political limelight. The answers and solutions offered by government could drastically alter the type and availability of health care as we know it today.

These same issues are a major challenge to your work as a hospital administrator. Working principally as a communicator and motivator of people, you must be in the front line of protectors of the advancements made in hospital management and health care.

Your skills as a communicator are essential to the building and continuation of your hospital's success. One industrial supervisor called it "The Velvet Boot Theory." He stated, "You must know how to give someone a kick in the pants without letting them feel the boot."

As motivator for a large group of people, project an inherent enthusiasm for your work and for the ultimate success of your hospital. Enthusiasm is contagious! Let those who implement your plans and policies *catch it*!

It is a fundamental rule that enthusiastic employees are more productive. Increased productivity, the key to cost control, begins with the enthusiastic leadership which only *you* can provide.

In this chapter, and throughout the book, our objective will be to assist you in focusing this vital force to enhance your hospital's operations. Knowing the basics of good management, plus effective budget planning, thorough knowledge of departmental operations, and all the other fundamentals of your job are *not* enough. If you fail to motivate department chiefs and employees, the medical staff, the board of trustees, and anyone else directly connected with your hospital's operations to new heights of excellence, your administrative efforts might end up in failure.

As cost containment and other factors presented by outside sources present an increasing influence on your hospital's operation, your communication abilities will become increasingly crucial. Every opportunity in which you can successfully motivate your employees to increase productivity and utilize their own innovative abilities to enhance the quality of their work will bring dividends toward your ultimate administrative goals.

The "Two Way" Administrative Street

To make the administrative process work at its finest, maintain open lines of communication with those who implement administrative policies. The "Closed Mind-Open Mouth" syndrome can have disastrous effects on the working relationships you want to develop.

Often, the people who are in direct daily contact with the departmental functions will have ideas which could prove beneficial to a hospital's operations. By encouraging these people to present their ideas, you may gain access to some excellent methods of enhancing efficiency.

A second benefit of this working relationship is that it improves the self-image of the employees and will invariably result in higher motivation and some noticeable increases in productivity.

If your hospital's financial position permits you to offer monetary rewards for better than average performance and achievement, you can really get your staff motivated.

Money "Talks" in Employee Relations

Though this term may seem like a time-worn cliché, it is nonetheless a "fact of life" to be reckoned with. Increasing employee productivity through traditional appeals for pride in a job well done no longer enjoys its previous success.

With the strong current monetary orientation, the fastest way to get a worker's attention is to reward productivity that helps to maintain your cost containment goals. As an example, if increased employee productivity for a department helps to cut operating expenses by 5 percent, passing 2 percent on to the department's staff would make good management sense. By getting employees to have a "stake" in the success of a department's operations, you can gain productivity without any large increase in supervisory effort.

If there is something to be gained by increased effort, employees will often monitor each other to get maximum output, particularly if the rewards are based on the total department performance, not on individual effort.

In a hospital where employees are unionized, this program might meet some initial resistance. For some reason, unions often take a dim view of incentive programs which are initiated by "management." This is based on two premises; (1) the belief that wage benefits should be increased based only on seniority, not on a worker's performance, and (2) the overriding fear that increased productivity, beyond a certain level, may threaten the existence of some employees' jobs.

If you can present this from the cost control angle, stressing that your primary objective is to gain a small measure of stability in escalating costs, you will probably gain their approval and enthusiastic support. If they believe that their jobs are not threatened by your actions, you can probably override concerns expressed in the first union premise.

The fact is that, given the economic conditions today and for the foreseeable future, the extra money which they might get from this type of program will overshadow their concerns for the underlying philosophy of the program.

CASE IN POINT: SHARED SAVING PLAN BRINGS DRAMATIC RESULTS FOR EUROPEAN HOSPITAL

As an example, a hospital in Europe sought to bring the costs for maintenance supplies into line. Suspecting that considerable waste occurred, they initiated a program similar to the one described above. It resulted in an immediate 10 percent reduction in supply use. The hospital passed along about 50 percent of the resulting savings to the department's staff, still leaving a 5 percent cost reduction for the hospital.

Winning employee support for this type of program is essential to its success. While enthusiastic support is the best, you can probably gain, at minimum, grudging concurrence by *implying* that staff reductions might be required if costs fail to be controlled by other means.

This "arm twisting" method is not advisable, except in cases where all other alternatives fail to get the desired results. This tactic can sometimes yield the unwelcome byproduct of a so-called wildcat strike, a walkout that can have disastrous repercussions on the hospital's productivity.

In some cases, when walkouts occur in vital service areas, it may force the hospital to close temporarily. This is particularly true if labor trouble strikes the dietary department.

CASE IN POINT: OHIO WALKOUT BRINGS EXTENDED REPERCUSSIONS

As an example, one Ohio hospital was forced to close for a week because dietary department personnel walked off their jobs in a dispute over new food handling equipment that reduced manpower needs by 20 percent.

Though the strike was resolved, the resulting community relations problem created by the forced closure prevented a return to normal operations for over six months.

This is the element that makes management decisions in the cost-containment realm so tricky to implement. On one hand, there can be substantial benefits derived from new equipment and procedures. However, if the hospital's staff adamantly resists the changes, the resulting crisis can thoroughly disrupt the normal flow of operations.

If there is any uncertainty within a community that a hospital will be able to serve its needs, this will have a definite effect on the institution's financial status—particularly so if there is more than one hospital in the area. The hospital displaying the greatest stability will gain the highest level of public confidence.

"Selling Benefits" in Administrative Policy

Because gaining staff approval and support is so important, make every effort to sell any proposed changes you might want to implement.

Action Idea: Before making any presentation, review all of the essential elements of your proposal with an emphasis on the real benefits your ideas will give to employees.

For instance, you might focus on getting the job done with less effort and greater efficiency. Everyone is interested in an easier method to get the job done. Whatever the proposal's benefits might be, you must be certain to address the employee's first natural question, "What's in it for me?"

If you can address this question effectively, you are unlikely to encounter any employee resistance. Because they are interested in continued job security and, as an offshoot of this, the success of the hospital, employees will enthusiastically implement your proposals. However, they must first be *convinced* of the proposal's merit.

This same principle applies to your relationship with the board of trustees. We definitely can't over-emphasize the importance of the dictum, "Do your homework." If you have a confident command of the facts pertaining to the proposal you are presenting, you are unlikely to meet major opposition (assuming the proposal is a reasonable one).

Any uncertainties which you state, or imply by your actions, will make your task of "selling" ideas more difficult. Therefore, it is vital that *you* are "sold" on the idea first. This confidence will readily project itself and make your job considerably easier.

Setting Realistic Goals

One of the greatest problems in this area is the tendency to have unrealistic expectations for the success of our plans. The myth of the "Overnight Success" is exactly that—a myth. Every worthwhile success that we experience is the result of cumulative effort over a longer period.

If your hospital is presently having major problems, it is tempting to raise the hopes of a fast turnaround in its fortunes. That's only natural! But the unvarnished truth is that such an occurrence is unlikely.

The central problem is not that your sights might be set too high. We believe that you should ultimately settle for nothing less than the best possible circumstances for your hospital. Rather, the problem is one of the time allotted for goal attainment.

We realistically can't expect major improvements to occur in a week or two, maybe not even in a month or two. Some major difficulties may take several years to be completely solved and eliminated from administrative planning.

This book itself is a prime example of elapsed time to "set the wheels in motion." More than six months passed from the time the idea for this book was conceived until the writing was begun. It passed through a number of phases to develop its ultimate shape.

The point that we wish to make is that you should not, to borrow an old cliché, "throw the baby out with the bath water," simply because an idea was not an instant success. If an idea's implementation shows progress toward the desired goal, give it some time to reach its peak potential.

By the same token, if an idea shows definite signs of proving counterproductive, you should scrap it without hesitation. Don't hang on to a "Pet Project," no matter how great it looked on paper, if its practical application does nothing to advance your hospital toward your administrative goals.

Admittedly, this might require a considerable degree of emotional detachment from you. But the inescapable fact is that masochism and effective hospital administration do not mix.

To sum up, setting realistic goals is primarily a matter of being realistic about the time required to achieve them. If you can exercise patience (and convince your Board of Trustees to do the same), almost any problem can be confronted and solved.

You may have to approach the problem in terms of short- and long-range goals. The short-range goals should be primarily directed to plugging some structural "leaks" and buy time for the implementation of your long-range objectives.

Whatever course of action you choose, you should definitely remember that "an optimistic captain can safely bring in a ship from the stormiest sea."

Mobilizing People: Some Final Thoughts

The key element to your success as a hospital administrator is *motivation*. The motivation level of your employees, physicians, department supervisors, and other personnel will largely determine the overall level of success your hospital will enjoy.

As stated in the beginning of this chapter, it is your *enthusiasm* that can turn the tide. If you are fired up, people around you will tend to be the same. This is the vital force that marks the successful people from the also-rans. If you do not settle for the average performance in yourself, your employees will be less likely to settle for it in themselves.

One noted public speaker called "average," "a case of mediocrity on a grand scale." You, as the leader, set the example for others to follow. Set your sights high! Believe in yourself!

This chapter, and those that follow, are basically designed to channel your creative energies and your present knowledge into the most constructive paths and methods to achieve the ultimate success for your hospital.

The decisive element that separates the successful facility from the unsuccessful is often creative stagnation, not a lack of basic knowledge. While we may, on occasion, find solutions that are so obvious that we wonder why the problem ever developed, the usual case requires "digging" to get the answers.

Today's modern hospital serves a two-fold purpose, both to serve the public's ultimate good: (1) it is a grand laboratory for today's great medical advancements, and (2) it is a sociological laboratory for the well-trained hospital administrator, reflecting, in a smaller sense, the great social forces outside the hospital.

Physicians, when faced with the rare, perplexing medical case, will sometimes opt for an attempted solution that is really "off the wall." The main criterion for the attempted solution is that it has the *possibility* of achieving its objectives.

You, like the physician, must occasionally make such assessments, with the only common caution that "no lasting harm is done to the patient." Without efforts of this type, very few of the advances your hospital enjoys today (in medicine or hospital management ideas) would be possible. Many of the ideas and solutions offered in this book were probably achieved in this way.

The true test of your administrative abilities and courage can be measured by your willingness to consider innovative ideas—and originate them! For many problems, a few minor changes—you might call them "course corrections"—may be all that is required. You may, however, face a problem that is singular to your hospital, one for which no set solution has been established.

After analyzing *all* possible solutions, including those of the off-the-wall variety, you must banish the paralysis of uncertainty, shedding it as a snake rids itself of its old skin, to permit the true growth potential within you and your hospital to be realized.

Bring these thoughts of expanded potential to your reading of subsequent chapters in this book. Study the ideas and examples we will present, using them as a springboard for your own resourcefulness and creativity.

Your knowledge and training are only the *foundation* for the structure of administrative success. Innovation is the key to survival—and to advancement—of the hospital health care delivery system. By joining us with this book, we believe that you have set out on the road to solving your hospital's problems and making your administrative efforts a resounding success!

Tested, successful organizational principles for your hospital

Your HOSPITAL'S ORGANIZATIONAL STRUCTURE is an important cornerstone in its overall success. Any major problem in this structure or inability to adapt as your hospital grows, will have an extremely detrimental impact on the institution's financial outlook.

This chapter will provide a "Back to Basics" review of the organizational structure for hospitals. As individual units, each hospital department may function reasonably well. Often, the real problems come from the *interrelationships* between various departments. If they can't work well together to form an efficient entity, nothing really works well.

We might easily compare this situation to that of the human anatomy, with each department being an important organ of the body. For example, your administrative office could be characteristically compared to the Brain. From your office, the signals go out to tell the hospital what must be accomplished.

By the same token, Financial Services might be described as the Heart of the hospital. Almost all of the institutional life blood must flow through this centrally important hospital department. If this department is not working efficiently, everything suffers.

This is the fundamental approach we must take to assure that your hospital operates at peak efficiency. Your diagnostic abilities must be so acute that you can readily spot the first signs of any impending illness in a department. Then, you can prescribe the necessary treatment before the entire hospital has a chance to suffer.

MINIMUM DEPARTMENTAL REQUIREMENTS

For a hospital to operate (or even be permitted to operate) most states require that seven essential departments be operated and maintained within generally accepted guidelines. These guidelines are set up as a standard for *minimum performance* for these departments.

The required departments are:

(1) A Dietary Department
(2) Medical Records Department
(3) Pharmacy or Drug Room
(4) Laboratories (Including Clinical Pathology)
(5) Radiology
(6) Emergency Service
(7) Medical Library

These seven departmental services provide the core for effective hospital operations. Without any one of them, the primary purpose of a hospital, providing top quality health care for its patients, would be seriously compromised.

Though our ultimate objective will be to obtain the maximum possible performance from each department in your hospital, we offer these guidelines as a foundation for your planning as well as a brief review of materials which you may have previously encountered.

Dietary Department

In any type of facility where people are housed for a period of days, weeks, or months, there is an obvious need to provide some sort of food accessibility.

The primary requirements for a dietary department are that it maintains an organized system with qualified personnel and is integrated with other departments in the hospital.

The main interconnection point for the dietary department is with the Medical Records Department. The medical staff needs dietary information as a basic part of its overall health care planning regimen for the patient.

So, if we were to make an interconnection chart for the Dietary Department, it would appear something like this:

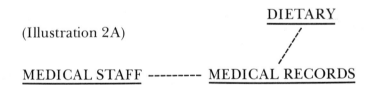

(Illustration 2A)

DIETARY

MEDICAL STAFF --------- MEDICAL RECORDS

If the communications links between these individual departments break down, some serious problems can result. For example, if a severe diabetic is placed on a general diet, the patient's blood sugar levels could rise to such levels as to trigger coma or even death. If such an error occurred, the hospital could be found liable of negligence and face severe financial losses (possibly exceeding levels of general liability protection).

An additional factor is the cost of inefficiency. Repeated communication failures can increase departmental expenses to an unacceptable level; meals for patients already discharged and no longer in the hospital, any special diets *not* required by a patient, etc. Though there are more possible examples, the general thrust of this idea is that we can't let things get out of control.

Further considerations in the dietary department would include adequate sanitation in the storage, preparation and distribution of food. A qualified dietician must be retained on a full-time or consultation basis, along with other administrative and technical personnel who are trained in their respective duties.

As mentioned earlier, a systematic record of diets must be maintained and correlated with the medical record department.

Finally, regular periodic conferences should be held within the department, and with other departments within the hospital, to be sure that adequate communications are maintained and efficiency enhanced.

Medical Records Department

This department is the meeting point for the elements involved in administering a hospital's patient health care services. As the limited diagram (see Illustration 2A) showed, information is funneled in from numerous sources to the Medical Records Department.

Here, as in no other area of hospital operations, the need for effective communications is crucial. Due to its relationship with a large number of departments, organization is crucial to maintaining a free flow of necessary information for health care services.

If a hospital's medical services were diagrammed according to the operational flow patterns, the medical records department would be the hub of a large, intricate operational wheel.

The central purpose of the department is, of course, to maintain medical records on every patient admitted for hospital care. These records must be kept confidential and retained for a period determined by your state's Statute of Limitations.

The department is also obligated to maintain an identification system for all records to allow speedy retrieval of a patient's record. Normally, the unit number system is preferred.

Adequate and qualified staffing is essential for this department. Because of the inherent complexity of its operations, created by the volume of records involved, the department may demand an increased staffing level to assure swift record delivery, enhancing care provided by the medical staff.

All clinical information pertaining to a patient should be centralized in the patient's record. Records should be categorized according to disease, operation, and physician involved, with updated entries (where required) completed by the conclusion of each business day. Any recognized indexing method may be used to serve the necessary indexing function.

The Joint Commission on Hospital Accreditation has stipulated that Standard Nomenclature be used as the nomenclature.

The most critical point in the operations of the Medical Records Department is its relationship with the hospital's medical and/or surgical staff. This subject will be discussed in greater detail later (see Chapter 9). For the present, it suffices to state that this is the center of a medical service's anatomy. Keeping this department at peak performance will help to assure the best possible health care delivery for your hospital's patients.

The Pharmacy

The hospital pharmacy or drug room plays a vital role in the treatment of patients, being central in the dispensation of all medications used in the hospital. Efficiency is vital here (see Chapter 15 for details) to maintain effective treatment programs.

The first essential requirement for the pharmacy is to have the direction of a registered pharmacist or, in the case of a drug room, competent supervision of the area's activities.

The pharmacy's facilities must provide adequate safeguards for secure storage, preparation, and dispensing of all medications. Competent personnel must be provided, based on the size and activity level of the department.

Federal and state laws require that detailed records be kept of every transaction made by the pharmacy, with correlation to other hospital records (where indicated).

All medications dispensed by the pharmacy must meet the standards set by the United States Pharmacopeia, National Formulary, or New and Non-official Drugs.

Special policies and security precautions are required to control the administration of toxic or dangerous drugs. Specific limitations of dosage and duration of use must be maintained. An example of such a medication is the painkiller morphine.

Because of the marked increase in illicit drug use, with a corresponding rise in thefts from hospital dispensaries, security measures must be taken to assure that a hospital's medications are always secure from this threat. Due to the remarkably high "street value" of controlled substances commonly found in hospitals, this problem is likely to increase in the future. (Solid security measures will also be discussed in Chapter 15.)

The final item in this generalized overview is the establishment of a medical staff oversight committee to confer with the pharmacist, helping him to formulate policies that are mutually beneficial to both pharmacy and medical staff.

Laboratories

Hospital laboratory services are divided into three general areas of expertise: (1) Clinical Pathology, (2) Blood Bank, and (3) Pathological Anatomy.

The clinical pathology function of a hospital lab should be maintained at a level which is adequate for the hospital's size and utilization demands. Basic minimum capabilities would include such pathological tests as chemistry, bacterial analysis, hematology (basic blood-testing capabilities), serum analysis, and clinical microscopy.

These services must be available at all times, with a 24-hours-a-day in-service or on-call status maintained to meet the needs of medical care in the hospital. To achieve this goal, adequate staffing levels must be maintained for both supervisory and working capacities.

Though standards for routine admission examinations should be determined by the medical staff, they must, at minimum, include a urinalysis and hemoglobin or hematocrit test.

Signed reports on lab test procedures and results should be filed with the patient's record, with duplicate copies maintained as a departmental record.

The essential function of the Blood Bank is to provide facilities for the safe procurement, storage and transfusion of blood. While some hospitals may have some entity nearby to handle this function, it is far preferable to maintain a blood bank facility on the hospital premises.

The third part, pathological anatomy, involves such details as tissue examinations after surgery and the autopsy studies. This service must be provided in any hospital where any surgery, however minor, is done.

All tissues removed during surgery should be sent for pathological examination, this being an effective review and monitoring process for the surgical staff. The extent of any pathological examination will be determined by tissue conditions revealed, as judged by the department's staff.

Signed tissue examination reports are to be filed with the patient's record, with duplicate copies being retained for departmental record keeping purposes.

Radiology

In most small and medium-sized hospitals, the Radiology department's activities are limited to the taking of x-rays and similar activities. In some hospitals, this department's functions are expanded to play a decisive role in cancer therapy with the use of radiation therapy.

The general requirement, however, is to maintain a radiology department that is in keeping with the needs displayed by the hospital's patient load.

The radiology department should be constructed with layout and equipment designed free of hazards for both patients and personnel. Adequate personnel for conducting and supervising radiological services must be provided.

"Reading" x-rays must be handled by a physician competent in this field, with signed reports handled in the same fashion as listed for other departments.

Emergency Service

Emergency service offers one of the greatest opportunities and challenges for the hospital's staff. The normal pace of hospital life is quickened as the virtual split-second precision of a hospital's emergency team goes into action. This is the area, according to some hospital administrators, that can be the greatest source of pride for the hospital.

Fundamentally, emergency service involves a written plan for handling care for mass casualties. Factory explosions, large residential fires, or multiple-collision freeway accidents are some examples of sources for the tough emergencies handled by this service.

The written plan should be practiced by key staff members at least twice a year. While these dress rehearsals offer a change of pace from standard hospital routine (employees sometime view it as school children see recess time), the key elements for preparation to meet a "real" emergency are always present.

The emergency service must meet the criteria of any other department regarding organization, qualified supervisory personnel, and integration with other hospital departments. Except in larger metropolitan hospitals, a standing emergency crew is not required to meet an area's needs.

Facilities should, however, be provided to assure prompt diagnosis and emergency treatment. Though rooms may or may not be set aside specifically for this purpose, they should be quickly convertible to handle a sudden influx of patients.

Hospitals providing emergency services must have adequate medical and nursing staff available at all times to meet the requirements.

Finally, though the pace of emergency service can be hectic, adequate medical records for every patient seen by the service must be kept. *

The Medical Library

This department usually serves both an internal and an external function in most hospitals. Technically, the purpose of the medical library is to support and enhance the available knowledge and reference sources for the hospital's medical and surgical staffs.

Therefore, the hospital must maintain a medical library that is sufficiently complex to meet the needs of its staff members. Textbooks and current periodicals are generally available and catalogued.

Trained personnel should be provided to insure efficient service to the medical staff. In addition to this vital function, the library can serve a public relations role by providing information to media people and others seeking specialized medical information. This role is especially important in areas where there is no access to university libraries on medical subjects.

Detailing Optional Medical Services

In addition to the seven services already mentioned with direct connection to the patient health care process, three other optional services can be provided to assist in patient care. They are: (1) Outpatient Department, (2) Rehabilitation Department, and (3) Medical Social Service Department.

Outpatient Department

In many hospitals, the outpatient department is a scaled down version of Emergency Services, geared to meet the needs of one or two patients at a time. The objective is to provide initial care, usually as a prelude to hospital admission.

---

* For additional information, see ¶5201 *et seq.*, Prentice-Hall *Hospital Cost Management Service.*

In some hospitals, this situation is changed to favor those that do not require around-the-clock acute hospital care, but require a specialized form of treatment. An example of this type of situation would be the use of kidney dialysis machines. Most patients would appear for six to eight hours on two or three days a week. These patients would not require continuous hospitalization, being free to go home after treatment.

In general terms, the structural requirements are similar for staffing, facilities, record keeping, and interdepartmental co-ordination as with other hospital departments.

A modification of this rule would occur in larger metropolitan hospitals where more detailed specialties are divided into smaller clinic-type settings. These are most often used with regional, rather than local, orientation in mind.

Rehabilitation Department

Rehabilitation services are an optional item that many hospitals choose to implement, if only on a limited basis. The most common of these services is the physical therapy department, covering accident or illness cases which have had a detrimental effect on limbs.

More refined, specialized services tend to be put together on a regional basis covering such areas as speech and occupational therapy, plus the brace and prosthetics (artificial limbs) shop.

The organization of a rehabilitation department is conducted comparably to other departments, with similar overall requirements.

Medical Social Services Department

This department, which could be called the Office of Patient Transition, plays a major role in cases where substantial physical and psychological adjustments are required of the patient and his (or her) family in the return to a home environment. This factor is particularly significant in cases where physical disability is prolonged or permanent.

In order for this department to fully meet its responsibility to physician, hospital, and patient, it must be well organized, under the direction of a qualified medical social worker, and firmly interconnected with other departmental activities within the hospital.

Facility requirements place a premium on patient accessibility and assured privacy for interviews. The department's location should also be conveniently located for access by the medical staff, along with the common space considerations for efficient departmental operations.

Records of case work must be kept. However, in contrast with other departments, these records should only be available to the professional personnel concerned with the case. The confidentiality of all social work cases must be assured!

The same departmental and interdepartmental communication links discussed for other departments also apply for the Medical Social Services Department.

Navigating a Stormy Sea

The preceding review of departmental functions was provided to refresh your memory of the basic functions and minimum performance standards that must be maintained for basic accreditation. As stated earlier, our objective is to get the best possible performance from each department of your hospital.

Unfortunately, external forces that are out of your control can play a major role in the success or failure of your hospital. As examples, government intervention in the forms of federal and state health care plans (Medicare, Medicaid, and similar programs) can sometimes bury a business office in paperwork. Efficient handling of this deluge can be a major asset to any hospital's profit picture.

Another problem area involves a hospital's utilization practices. In some cases, this can be an area of stormy confrontation between 1) the hospital's need to get the best possible efficiency from its hospital space, and 2) patients' needs, either physical or psychological. This area demands a balance between the humanitarian objectives of management and the cold business realities of operating a hospital in today's complex financial times.

In larger hospitals, the utilization problem is complicated somewhat by the clearer divisions between medical and surgical services. If, for example, a hospital's medical service has a shortage of beds to meet its needs while the surgical service has a surplus, it is the administrator's duty to reallocate the bed capacities for each service.

By adjusting the allocations of hospital space to reflect fluctuating levels of demand, the administration can get maximum usage of every hospital bed. That is the primary objective. Every empty bed presents a negative cost factor to the hospital.

This factor does not customarily affect the smaller hospital where such clear-cut division between the medical and surgical services does not exist. Rather, the 100-bed or less semi-rural or rural hospital often runs an informal arrangement, concentrating surgical cases into a small number of rooms, shrinking or expanding their number as the need arises.

In an area that does not support a steady flow of surgical cases, this appears to be the wisest course of action. This prevents empty beds because the available patient's condition does not fit the "set-aside" description for the available bed.

By the same token, a hospital can be *over-used* to the point that flexibility to meet emergency situations is restricted. The common criterion is that occupancy exceeding 85 percent could place a hospital's response capability into serious jeopardy.

Maintaining this balance can cause serious problems in some medical cases where the patient's condition is marginal; the patient may be too well to need acute hospital care, yet not well enough to be returned home. In many areas, particularly those with high concentrations of senior citizens, the Extended Care capacity is woefully inadequate to meet the demands.

This situation is complicated by the fact that many areas depend on county or state-financed facilities to provide the vast majority of this care. While the economic conditions affecting government expenditures may prevent further investments, the need continues to increase.

CASE IN POINT: FRUSTRATION IN EXTENDED CARE

One county Extended Care Facility in Michigan had a waiting list exceeding 100 patients needing care. This would have permitted utilization for twice the number of patients currently housed in the facility. Because funding is not available, the situation (at the time of this writing) remains unresolved.

Finding the Balance

The preceding case history clearly illustrates the problem that this situation creates. Even in areas where private enterprise has provided adequate facilities to meet the need, government funding (or the lack of it) plays a crucial role in the levels of care these patients receive.

As one administrator explained it: "We face the situation of having to form a budget in July and finding out how much money we'll get in October. This is no way to run a hospital."

Escalating costs, along with an increasing public mood to limit government spending, appear to be compounding this crisis. The problem extends itself into every area of hospital and medical management, placing a serious cloud over the training of future doctors and nurses.

As one college nursing school coordinator put it, "If any of the current tax reduction programs under consideration pass the legislature, or are approved by voters, we might as well close our doors. We are finished! We may not be able to see our current classes through to graduation, even with the present situation."

No area of hospital administration is immune from the influence of government whims, provided that even a small portion of a hospital's funding comes from a federal or state agency. Though this problem does have some bearing on the privately owned or community acute care hospital, it has an even more devastating impact on the long-term, extended care facility.

One possible answer to this problem would be to have closer coordination between the state and federal budgetary processes and those of the dependent institutions. If the adjustments are completely one-sided, with the burden falling on the health care administrator, it could create a temporary (but potentially disastrous) financial crisis.

For example, if a hospital's budgetary process was to be finalized in July for the upcoming year, and the state's budgetary year begins in October, this would leave a three-month adjustment period.

The most obvious solution to this problem is probably the most difficult to achieve. If a hospital's budget was changed to meet the governmental budget period, all that would be required is a request for 15 months worth of allocation instead of 12 to bridge the financial gap. Right?

Not likely! Government agencies probably would strongly resist a 25 percent funding increase, above the normal requirements of inflation, without regard to the nobility of its purpose. If the budget period adjustment is made without a corresponding adjustment in the funding levels, the financial shortages could become quite severe.

Clearly, the answer to this problem is a cooperative effort between government agencies and the health care providers. In the final analysis, government social programs designed to provide health care for the poor must be constructed to meet the dual needs of both the patient and the health care provider.

Your role is to communicate and fight for the needs of your hospital. Present your case to those responsible for financial decisions on the federal, state, and local levels. Get the attention of your senators and representatives. "Bend an ear" or do some gentle "arm twisting" if you must. But be certain that they recognize the serious nature of hospital funding problems created by poorly constructed government social programs.

No hospital is financially equipped to dispense an endless stream of charity to the community. The inherent problems of government funding must be met head-on. There is no choice! The ultimate benefactors will be the financially indigent patients your hospital serves.

Insurance Programs: Public and Private

In the early and mid-1960's, the issue of government-sponsored health insurance programs for the public was raised under the banner of Lyndon Johnson's Great Society. As a direct result, the funding of health care for the elderly was drastically altered by the implementation of the Medicare insurance programs.

At the time of this writing, this same issue is being raised again, expanding the national "Medicare idea" to cover all United States citizens. While the projected paper work for hospitals probably would not be noticeably greater than for private insurers, the specter of major government regulation of fee and pricing structures could present a major problem for hospital administrators.

Though this would serve as a form of "financial insurance," assuring that a hospital would get paid for every patient it treats, the increasing role of government in the administrative decision-making process would be inevitable. Just as private insurers now make their recommendations on hospital size, expansion proposals, etc., the federal government's intervention into this process could carry the weight of law; i.e., if the National Insurer decides that you don't need ten new beds in your hospital, you won't be allowed to build them.

By the same authority, if they decide that one part of your hospital's operations needs to be upgraded, they might force the issue on you, leaving you to worry about how the project will be financed. As is characteristic with government programs, they will often mandate a certain standard to be followed without providing the necessary financial assistance to meet their objectives.

In addition, as your past encounters with the current Medicare program would show, they maintain certain standards regarding "fair and reasonable charges" for hospital services, not taking into account the local cost variations which you must live with daily.

Private insurers that offer "supplemental"coverage to Medicare beneficiaries base their payments on the amounts that the Medicare administration approves. In this case, government standards are applied to all insurance coverage provided to the patient.

In Chapter 5, dealing with Financial Services, we will get into greater detail about the specifics on dealing with government forms, private insurance paper work, etc. At this point, it suffices to state that the inherent policies of public and private insurers have a substantial impact on the direction of your hospital's activities. Being in charge of the "collective purse," they can either reward or punish you, depending on how they view the direction of your administration.

Whether we like it or not, these controls tend to have a restrictive effect on a hospital's ability to expand or improve its current services. As you will note in the next section of this chapter, this factor could make a hospital uncompetitive in providing some forms of health care.

Prepayment Plans

One of the most controversial, but fast-growing, methods of financing health care is the prepayment plan. Under this system, doctors and other health care providers are *paid for keeping people well.*

As such, the increasing popularity of the system could, in the long term, result in decreased utilization of hospital services. With an emphasis on prevention, the physicians treating participating patients will garner a larger portion of the available money from these programs.

Additionally, as noted in an article by Jeff Goldsmith in the *Harvard Business Review,* there is an increasing trend toward in-office or outpatient treatment of many medical problems. Because of the increasing financial resources that many physicians now have, they can effectively compete with hospital services, frequently underselling the hospital.

When the finite financial sources of the prepayment plans are added to the picture, it is clear that these physicians will opt to gain the entire fee, not sharing it with the hospital. This factor, along with others designed to reduce or limit in-patient hospital utilization, may prove to have a detrimental effect on the financial prospects of many hospitals.

A study conducted by the Blue Cross insurance group reveals the true extent of this "siphoning off" from the normally expected inpatient hospital usage. According to the study, in a period from 1968 to 1978, an 18.6 percent decline in hospital inpatient days was registered. Yet, in the same period, a 137.6 percent increase in outpatient visits for Blue Cross subscribers was registered.

With this trend so dramatically illustrated among the traditionally insured population, the extensive use of HMO's (Health Maintenance Organizations, as prepayment plans are popularly referred to) present a direct competitive challenge to the hospitals.

The basic philosophy of HMO programs is that a set figure for health care is calculated per patient annually regardless of whether or not the individual is hospitalized. This policy makes it financially more lucrative to keep the patient out of the hospital.

As health care programs become increasingly oriented toward preventing patient hospitalization, the competition for available patients will become more intense. In some areas with a higher concentration of facilities to available patient population, hospital closures have resulted. In other cases, two or more hospitals have merged to restrict administrative and employment costs, making the resulting health care provider more competitive in the shrinking health care market. *

The Challenge Ahead

The real "clincher" to this problem is the rapid advance of medical science. As new technological developments occur at a rapid rate, this presents another problem for you, the hospital administrator. On one side, you are obliged to observe the financial constraints presented by a potentially reduced health care market. On the other, you must keep your hospital up to date if you hope to keep your hospital attractive to the medical profession.

A hospital that is woefully behind the current medical and surgical technologies will have severe problems in keeping its current staffs in place. From the viewpoint of future hospital security, this problem is even more acute. If a hospital does not maintain modern standards, it has little hope of attracting new doctors to fill the normal attrition that would occur in any medical or surgical staff.

To meet the challenge of adequate hospital utilization, service diversification appears to be one of the potential solutions to be explored.

CASE IN POINT: MIDWEST HOSPITAL EFFECTIVELY ULTIMATES NEW SOURCES FOR NEW PATIENTS

At one metropolitan hospital in the Midwest, an extensive outpatient program has handled more than 220,000 outpatient visits annually. In addition, their emergency room services have handled 80,000 visits.

As a result, this hospital has gained more than 95 percent of its hospital admissions from these two sources.

Though this method does offer considerable merit in the patient acquisition process, some inherent cost factors in maintaining such programs could dampen your enthusiasm for their implementation.

Because overhead for outpatient services has risen comparably with that of inpatient hospital care, the hospital outpatient department may still be at a considerable competitive disadvantage to similar services provided by physicians' offices.

Later in this book, we will discuss some of the cost factors on which any implementation decisions are to be made. With the current sentiments of public and

---

* See also ¶3401 *et seq.,* Prentice-Hall *Hospital Cost Management Service.*

private insurers favoring outpatient procedures, many hospitals may have little choice but to implement or expand outpatient services. Unless they do so, the financial viability of the health care providers may be in serious jeopardy.

The only dark cloud on this horizon comes from the federal regulations governing reimbursements from Medicare and Medicaid programs. They authorize payment based on cost or charges, whichever is lower. Based on their formulas for "fair and reasonable charges," a hospital could be required to perform some services at a financial loss.

Firm Hand at the Helm

With the great challenges to a hospital's future, today's administrator needs some essential background to cope with the problems his job presents.

Fundamentally, the hospital administrator must have a considerable degree of business acumen. Despite the human services angle of hospital management, it is nonetheless a business. As such, some decisions (if not most) must be made on the basis of profitability for the institution. At the minimum, financial loss must be prevented.

For this reason, we recommend that *every* hospital administrator have a background in business administration. This should be coupled with a firm foundation in medical administration, the application of business principles to the clinical setting.

Over the years, hospital administration has evolved into a separate, distinct profession. As a result, several university programs in hospital administration have become available in the United States. As the need for specialized administrative planners increases, in direct proportion to the challenges to hospital systems, more programs of this type will probably result.

Clearly, the future trend points toward the employment of specialized administrators for most hospitals. While this does not imply that current administrators without such training will be rendered immediately obsolete, the increasing challenges of the field would seem to favor the specialist.

Hospital Organization: Some Final Thoughts

Over the length of this chapter, we have sought to present a reasonably accurate picture of the total challenge in an administrator's task. By necessity, this picture has been a "rough sketch" without the subtle, intricate details of departmental operations.

In the chapters which follow, we will present the finer details which will convert this rough sketch into a Master Design for hospital administration. Regardless of your present background, we are certain that the problem-solving materials which will be presented can have a positive impact on the medical, scientific, and financial integrity of your hospital.

Up to now, we have presented only the essential "skeleton" for a successful hospital. Now it is time to put "meat on the bones," through the next 20 chapters, to create the living entity you want your hospital to be.

The medical core of hospital management

ONE FUNDAMENTAL AREA OF HOSPITAL MANAGEMENT deserves considerable attention: development of a solid, efficient, and cohesive medical staff for an acute care hospital. No hospital can render effective care if inadequate staffing is a glaring weakness in the management plan.

The unspoken reality of the physicians' power to determine a hospital's course should never be underestimate or minimized. The physician is the ultimate judge as to a hospital's utilization levels. He decides when a patient is to be admitted and discharged from the hospital.

For this reason, some hospitals retain staff physicians (on salary) to augment doctors maintaining private practices outside the hospital. Another trend showing administrative awareness of this problem is for hospitals to provide office space within their buildings for physicians' private practices.

As discussed in Chapter 2, regarding the increasing inclination of physicians to compete with hospitals for certain services, the physicians' presence within the hospital may tend to discourage this practice. The doctor who is given office facilities for minimal charge might feel indebted to the hospital, to refer any but the most minor cases for in-hospital treatment. There is also the underlying psychological control factor, though unspoken, that if a physician begins to compete with the hospital on services, he may be asked to vacate his office facilities and seek others outside the hospital.

The financial benefits of an in-hospital office are usually sufficient to make a doctor hesitant to risk such a result. The reduced overhead keeps the profits of the private practice at an acceptably high level, much better than if he were required to maintain his practice elsewhere.

As you can see, the relationship between a hospital's administrative office and its medical staff can sometimes become a psychological tug of war. If the inherent benefits of playing ball with Administration are sufficient, there shouldn't be too much difficulty in getting the medical staff to work toward mutually beneficial goals.

The balance of this two-part chapter examines in further detail the organizational aspects of developing a medical staff. The second part will get into the nuts and bolts of an effective administration-medical staff relationship, with emphasis on maintaining close ties between the two departments to insure the future financial and medical integrity of your hospital.

PART 1 — HOW TO ORGANIZE AN EFFECTIVE AND EFFICIENT MEDICAL STAFF

Basically, the organizational structure of a hospital's medical staff is designed to insure that the inherent responsibilities of an institution's physicians to its patients, administration, and the governing body are met in a satisfactory fashion.

Maintaining a high standard of medical care for the hospital must be the medical staff's primary concern. In order to meet this primary objective, the staff organizational structure must carry out the following six essential duties:

(1) Make recommendations to the Administration and to the governing body of the hospital regarding staff appointments and hospital privileges.
(2) Conduct continuing analytical review of all clinical work and practices done within the hospital.
(3) Actively support individual members of the medical staff and hospital policies.
(4) Insure that adequate medical records are kept.
(5) Procure autopsies and monitor the minimum standards (20 percent to 25 percent of all hospital deaths) for such activities.
(6) Conduct consultations.

Staff Member Responsibility

In order for the medical staff organizational concept to work at all, some fundamental objectives must be met by each member of the staff.

First and foremost, the physician's responsibility is to the patients under his care. Clearly, the doctor must provide the best care that his intellectual capabilities and the physical limitations of the hospital will allow.

Second, the physician is responsible to the inner organization of the medical staff, subject to the adopted standards, rules and regulations set up by the Staff bylaws. While this situation requires a considerable amount of self-monitoring (a problem we'll discuss in a moment) and monitoring the activities of his colleagues, this mechanism can *usually* be depended upon to maintain *minimum standards* for hospital medical care.

Third, there is the responsibility to the governing body of the hospital. The responsibility is primarily to assist in attaining and maintaining the goals set forth by the governing body and administration of the hospital.

Staff "Politics" and Medical Standards

One substantial problem of the self-monitoring process for the medical profession lies in the considerable reluctance to step on the toes of any individual members. Unless the violations of medical procedure or ethics are so glaring as to attract considerable public attention, the profession's natural inclination is to brush it under the carpet. They clearly operate under the premise, "Who knows when it could happen to me?"

As the old saying about stone throwing in glass houses implies, this hesitancy has much to do with the individual physician's recognition of his own human frailties. It also means that you, as a hospital administrator, must be vigilant concerning the standards of your hospital. You can't become overly reliant upon the internal monitoring system set up by your medical staff.

This subject is brought up here as a matter which might merit some concern, not as an indictment of the medical profession. The most effective method of assuring that adequate standards are met is through the cooperative efforts of both you and the medical staff.

With both sides having one eye on the other, the high standards normally expected by the consuming public can be maintained.

Internal Organization for the Medical Staff

The backbone of any staff organization mechanism starts with the established chain of command which is implemented. A hospital's medical staff is, of course, no exception to this rule.

By necessity, a medical staff must be organized along authoritative lines. Someone must be the final point of authority, the decision maker on the staff. Each of the offices on the medical staff should be filled to make the mechanism work at its best. This can be accomplished by appointment from the administrative level or through election by the medical staff members.

Because of the clear duty to maintain medical standards within the hospital, staff officers should have the authority to enforce staff rules, differentiate hospital privileges, conduct disciplinary actions (when necessary), and to make definitive recommendations to the governing body regarding appointments to and terminations from the hospital's medical staff.

Under the commonly held concepts of medical staff organization, one physician holds a dominant role on the staff, often with the designation of Chief of Staff. Under the Chief's direction, eight committees serve the hospital in an advisory capacity. These committees, though operating interdependently, have separate and distinct functions within the hospital management organization.

The eight committees are: (1) the Executive Committee, (2) the Joint Conference Committee, (3) the Credentials Committee, (4) the Medical Records Committee, (5) the Tissue Committee, (6) the Medical Audit Committee, (7) the Infection Committee, and (8) the Utilization Committee.

Chief of Staff

At the head of this diverse organizational mechanism is one physician, designated as the Chief of Staff. While this designation is often given to one individual, on a rotating basis, for a one-year period, the interests of continuity would probably be better served by a two to three-year period for this position.

Regardless of the method your hospital employs for this position, there is the fundamental question of the desirable qualities for the best possible chief of staff. What qualities do you look for?

Most important: The chief of staff must have a high level of leadership capability. A first-class Milquetoast without even a grain of assertiveness just will not make the grade at this position.

Along with the leadership qualification, the prospective chief of staff should be an active member of the hospital's medical staff for a minimum of five years, care for the largest percentage of his patients within the hospital where he will be Chief, have membership on one of the eight standing committees for a three-year period (with chairmanship for one year), and command the respect of his colleagues inside and outside the hospital.

A valuable adjunct to these qualifications is the ability to be a diplomat. Since he often serves in a liaison capacity between the medical staff and the governing body and administration of the hospital, his abilities can be put to a severe test. With the powerful interests of the medical staff on one side, he must bridge the chasm between the two different viewpoints, to their mutual benefit.

From the authority standpoint, the chief of staff is responsible for the smooth running of the medical staff. Either directly, or through the delegation of portions of this function, the Chief must maintain firm, careful supervision over every aspect of the clinical work done within the hospital. Except where administrative and clinical interests merge, the Chief is "King of the Mountain." In the clinical area of hospital management, the chief of staff's authority reigns supreme.

Within the chain of command, your relationship with the chief of staff must, by necessity, be a fairly smooth one. If things break down in this area, the entire range of medical care will be adversely affected. The chief of staff will be your link to the various committees that facilitate the smooth operations of the entire medical staff.

The Executive Committee

This committee serves as the focal point of the entire committee process for the medical staff. As such, the executive committee has the broadest range of authority of any internal committee within the hospital.

With the expressed authorization of the medical staff, it coordinates policies and departmental activities for the entire staff, serves in an oversight capacity for the other standing committees of the medical staff, and is the primary authority for disciplinary actions taken against any individual staff member.

Membership in this committee usually consists of the chief of staff, the secretary, and a minimum of three active members of the hospital's medical staff. This membership is by election or appointment, usually not to exceed a one-year term.

Meetings are normally conducted once a month, more often if staff business so dictates, with written minutes containing time of meeting, members present and absent, and details of any items of business decided at the meeting. Also included would be any reports or recommendations to be made to the medical staff and the hospital's governing body. This written report of the committee meeting must be signed by the chairman of the executive committee.

Joint Conference Committee

The Joint Conference Committee serves in a special liaison capacity within the medical staff committee framework, bridging the communication void between the medical staff, the administrator's office, and the governing board of the hospital. In this capacity, the joint conference committee is the forum where ideas, policies, programs, and problems which merit consideration by both clinical and administrative management structures are formulated.

The composition, responsibilities, and actions of the joint conference committee are usually spelled out in the bylaws governing the medical staff. As a general rule, this committee is composed of three doctors from the medical staff and three members of the governing board. The administrator serves, usually, as secretary for the group.

Tenure on the joint conference committee, applying to both medical staff members and board members, is generally limited to one year. By maintaining a fairly frequent turnover, a deeply entrenched power structure in this vital area is avoided.

The method of committee record keeping is similar to that discussed in the section on the Executive Committee.

One area in which the joint conference committee is particularly important is in handling appeals of any disputed rulings made by other medical staff committees. This appeal authority should be granted to the joint conference committee through the bylaws and regulations governing the medical staff.

Any recommendations made in the joint conference committee should, of course, be passed on to the entire medical staff and to the governing board for their disposition.

The Credentials Committee

The primary function of the credentials committee is to serve as a screening body for applicants to positions on the medical staff, as well as to review the suitability of present members for continued tenure.

With direct responsibility to the executive committee, the credentials committee is generally composed of three to five members of the active and consulting staff. In larger hospitals, this may be varied to include a member of each specialty offered in the hospital.

Members of the credentials committee are elected, or in some cases appointed, by the chief of staff or the executive committee. The usual term of committee membership is one year.

The business of the credentials committee is usually conducted in a formally prescribed manner. Any applicants subject to review by the committee normally submit a written application on a prescribed form, stating full details of their qualifications for the appointment; education, experience, and interests are all pertinent information in this area.

Applicants' information should normally be supported by two or more written references from physicians known to members of the committee. Also, any character references that the applicant might wish to offer can be considered.

When this information is given to the committee, they will verify, or ask the administrator to do so, that the applicant being considered has the necessary educational and licensing credentials to practice the area of medicine or surgery for which application is made. Any documentation obtained as verification should be maintained in the personnel file for the doctor retained on the hospital's staff. Also, the file should include a signed statement by the applicant stating that he (or she) will abide by the bylaws and regulations established for the medical staff of the hospital.

The lines of communication from the Credentials Committee include responsibility to the Executive Committee and regular communications with the hospital's administrator; it also passes its recommendations to the governing board for final action.

When the credentials committee has made its final decision on an applicant, they pass this on to the Administrator. The administrator is responsible for making the presentation to the governing board.

The governing board, in turn, either accepts or rejects the applicant after consultation with the joint conference committee. If the physician is appointed, the administrator processes the appointment and notifies the applicant of the action in writing.

As outlined for the executive committee earlier, similar record-keeping for the committee's activities is required here.

The credentials committee's oversight function is a vital link in assuring that the minimum standards for hospital accreditation (from a medical and surgical viewpoint) are attained and maintained.

The Medical Records Committee

In the area of day-to-day quality control over a hospital's clinical activities, no medical staff committee holds a greater share of the responsibility than the Medical Records Committee. By a thorough review of patient records, this committee monitors the professional activities of every member of the hospital's staff, making certain that the highest standards of professionalism are met. In addition, this review process provides a high level of legal protection to hospital, staff members, and patients alike.

Membership in this vital committee should have a minimum of three active members from the medical staff, appointed for a minimum one-year term by the executive committee.

In conducting their mandated review process, the medical records committee works closely with the medical records librarian. The librarian's job is to conduct the clerical functions of the task, leaving the committee with only the responsibility of judging the quality of care based on the documentation presented by the librarian.

One of the primary functions of the medical records committee is to be sure that adequate records are kept of all clinical activities conducted in the hospital. For this reason, this committee should have the authority to approve new forms, delete unnecessary ones, and make recommendations on the record-keeping procedures to insure that the highest standards in patient care, professional education, and medical staff functioning are maintained.

Patient records, according to customary committee standards should include each of the eight following specific items:

(1) Summary Sheet.
(2) Patient History.
(3) Physical Examination.
(4) Laboratory Reports.
(5) Physicians' Orders.
(6) Progress Notes.
(7) Graphic Record.
(8) Nurses' Notes.

These eight items comprise the recognized minimum of information required by every patient who has been hospitalized, regardless of the time period involved.

In cases involving more extensive care, surgical procedures, or the death of a patient, a far more involved list of forms and records is utilized to be certain that the legally and scientifically valid informational system is adequate. Some of these additional records might include:

 (1) Consultations.
 (2) Labor Record.
 (3) Birth Certificate.
 (4) Release from Responsibility for Abortion.
 (5) Authority to Operate.
 (6) Anesthesia Record.
 (7) Operation Record.
 (8) Tissue Report.
 (9) Report of Infection.
(10) Death Certificate.
(11) Authority for Autopsy.
(12) Autopsy Report.
(13) Survey of Operative Mortality Case.
(14) Survey of Maternal Mortality Case.
(15) X-ray reports.
(16) Electrocardiography Report.
(17) Urology Report.
(18) Release from Responsibility for Discharge.
(19) Others, as instructed.

Based on the 20 or more reports that could potentially find their way into a patient's record, the total picture of a hospital's quality of medical and surgical care can be obtained. If each member of the medical and surgical staff makes sure his records are kept current, the medical records committee's job is made relatively simple.

This committee serves as the hospital's "insurance policy" that adequate standards are being met. If you, as administrator, maintain an effective liaison with this committee, you can be reasonably assured that the fundamental standards for hospital care will be met.

The Tissue Committee

Somewhat similar to the functions of the medical records committee, the Tissue Committee serves as the monitoring point for the surgical procedures conducted within the hospital. Here, the primary liaison point comes between this committee and the hospital's staff pathologist.

Surgery, unlike general medicine, tends to be more specific in its objectives. Based on the human tissue removed during surgery, a subjective analysis of the merits (or demerits) of any given procedure can be made. This analytical process is the primary reason for the existence of a tissue committee in a surgical hospital.

The tissue committee, whether appointed by the chief of staff or by the executive committee, should contain at least one surgeon and the hospital's pathologist. The total membership of the tissue committee should be a minimum of three, each member being appointed for a minimum one-year term.

At minimum, meetings of the tissue committee should be conducted monthly, more frequently if surgical business warrants it. Minutes of committee meetings, kept and written by the medical records librarian or the medical secretary, serving as secretary for the committee, are kept for all committee functions.

Also included in the committee secretary's functions is maintaining a running report on surgical success rates and related data for committee analysis and comment. These would include appropriate items from the records presented for review by the medical records committee.

Records for all surgical patients discharged from the hospital subsequent to the last committee meeting are made available for tissue committee scrutiny. For the sake of impartiality, the attending surgeon on any case is not permitted to review his own records. These are assigned to another member of the committee.

An overall analysis of surgical results is compiled for each individual member of the hospital's surgical staff. When appropriate, these reports and tissue committee recommendations are passed on to the executive committee. None of these review reports, or the resulting recommendations, are to be included in the official record for any individual patient.

The Medical Audit Committee

In some hospitals, serving the interests of greater efficiency, the Medical Audit Committee becomes a form of consolidation between two previously mentioned committees, medical records and tissue.

In this capacity, the functions of the medical audit committee would be the combined responsibilities already discussed for the medical records committee and the tissue committee.

If this mode is adopted, membership in the medical audit committee should have a minimum of three, representing the departments of Medicine, Obstetrics, and Surgery. Larger hospitals might wish to include a representative from each of the hospital's specialties.

Appointments to the medical audit committee, like those of the two component committees this one might replace, would be made by the chief of staff or by the executive committee. The general length of term is usually one year, though members may serve for three to six-month periods, in rotation.

Meetings are held monthly, more often if necessary, with functions and reporting mechanisms similar to those outlined for other committees in this chapter. This committee is ultimately responsible to the executive committee and to the chief of staff.

The Infection Committee

The Infection Committee is one of the broadest-based committees in the medical organizational structure of the hospital. Containing representatives from the medical and surgical staffs, the nursing staff, the pathology department, the local health department, and other departments (as indicated by need), this committee serves a vital monitoring function over hospital activities to reduce incidences of infection in patients and hospital personnel.

In this capacity, the infection committee is responsible for developing a detailed hospital policy for infection control, as well as periodically reviewing it to judge its adequacy for changing conditions.

The policy structure instituted for infection control is, by necessity, relatively complex. Here, in brief, are some elements of an effective infection control policy. These 14 points of policy, though varied somewhat according to need, form the cornerstone for effective hospital infection control.

Elements for Effective Hospital Infection Control

(1) Continuing orientation and education of all staff members on effective infection prevention, identification, control, and management procedures.

(2) Detailed review of all infection cases.

(3) An effective mechanism for tracing the source and causes of any infections occurring within the hospital.

(4) Availability of lab facilities to conduct periodic evaluations and cultures on infant formulas, autoclaves, and water sterilizers. This would include a detailed microbiological analysis.

(5) Admitting physician must notify committee of any infection present in patient, if known, upon admission to the hospital.

(6) A detailed policy to control the use of any antibiotics in the hospital, prohibiting their use as a preventive measure when no infection is present. This would also include cultures and sensitivity tests in infected cases prior to

administering any antibiotics. (Routine use of antibiotics tends to increase incidents of infection.)

(7) Enforcement of proper hygienic procedures, including proper handwashing and scrubbing practices, gown and mask techniques, materials and instruments packaging, packing of the autoclaves, and appropriate procedures for dressing-cart usage.

(8) Maintenance and proper use of isolation facilities and techniques.

(9) Effective and efficient housekeeping procedures to assure that proper standards for cleanliness in all areas of the hospital are maintained; this is the surest method of restricting the spread of infection.

(10) Monitoring all dietary and food handling procedures, refrigeration, ice bins, dishwashing, and proper disinfection procedures for all contaminated utensils.

(11) Monitoring laundry practices.

(12) Implementing appropriate safeguards on all air conditioning, ventilation, and heating systems for a hospital, with positive air pressure for operating, delivery, recovery, emergency, newborn nursery, and central supply rooms. Negative air pressure should be maintained for isolation, anesthesia storage, autopsy, laundry and soiled linen rooms, kitchen, toilets and bathrooms. The recirculation of air should be prohibited in the surgical suite, obstetrical suite, emergency room, isolation, formula preparation units, nurseries, pathology, virus and bacteriological labs, media rooms, autopsy and dark rooms, laundry and soiled linen rooms, kitchens, toilets and bathrooms.

(13) Establishment of proper handling procedures and disposal techniques for wastes and the excretions of sputum, feces and urine, and environmental wastes of dressings, food, and floor sweepings.

(14) Maintenance of effective traffic controls and visiting rules in all areas of the hospital, with particular emphasis on the operating room, nursery, obstetrical, and isolation areas.

Though the dangers of infection will probably always be present in the hospital environment, the implementation of these 14 specific control areas in a concerted fashion should effectively minimize the dangers to both patients and hospital personnel.

This is the primary responsibility of the infection committee. Encouraging the proper discharge of its function will assure you of the maximum safety and efficiency for your hospital.

The Utilization Committee

In the area of total hospital resource management, no single committee or authority wields greater power on the lives of patients and doctors alike than the hospital's Utilization Committee. As the monitoring entity for usage levels of hospital resources, it is the utilization committee's function to be certain that appropriate resource utilization levels, neither too high nor too low, are maintained.

Because either extreme can have an adverse effect on the quality and cost of the patient care delivered to the community, the effects of this committee's actions on public relations, personnel and facilities costs, benefits of prepayment plans and other hospital care financing options, and the general public perceptions of the hospital and its medical and surgical staffs can never be underestimated.

The utilization committee normally consists of appointed representatives from the medical staff, a minimum of four, with assistance from the medical records librarian and administration. Meetings, as with other hospital committees, should be held monthly (at minimum) to review records regarding the use of facilities.

Though many portions of the utilization committee's function are monitored by other internal committees of the medical staff, this separate committee is a requirement of the Joint Commission on Accreditation of Hospitals as well as for participation in the federal Medicare program. (If, as alluded to earlier in this book, National Health Insurance becomes a reality, the utilization committee will play an even greater role in the hospital's overall functions.)

For each hospital admission, a hospital's utilization committee must have established criteria to cover the following five areas:

(1) Conditions for patient admission.
(2) Standards for diagnostic procedures.
(3) Complications affecting length of stay.
(4) The customary length of hospitalization for any given illness.
(5) Indications for discharge.

From the broad range viewpoint, the utilization committee has ten general goals in the area of resource management. They are:

(1) Reducing the number of excessive patient hospitalization days.
(2) Restricting unnecessary admissions and preventing over-utilization of ancillary services.
(3) Maintaining close communications links between the medical staff, administration, and the hospital social service department.
(4) Maintaining heightened awareness of over-utilization's effects on prepayment plans and public and private insurance carriers.
(5) Enhancing quality and speed of medical charting.
(6) Reviewing, as needed, of the admission and discharge procedures.
(7) Reducing pre-operative hospitalization.
(8) Improving procedures for emergency admissions.
(9) Rapid transfer from one medical or surgical service to another, as indicated by patient's condition.
(10) Improving procedures, where necessary, for handling disposition problems and transition difficulties for discharges of long-stay cases.

In reviewing the goals and standards that are the province of the utilization committee, the criteria that each hospital's committee sets for its medical staff have a broad-range impact on the quality and quantity of hospital care that will be rendered. Because of this fact, it is imperative that a hospital's administration take an extremely active role in this particular area.

Without your active participation in the actions of the utilization committee, some administrative objectives could be scuttled by committee actions.

The Hospital Medical Staff: A Final Review

Medical staff organization, while generally the same for most hospitals, must, in the minute details, become tailored to the individual needs of each hospital. The medical staff requirements for a general care community hospital are substantially different from those for a hospital that has a substantial number of critically ill patients. As an example, a hospital that conducts open heart surgery has substantially different requirements, from a medical staff viewpoint, from a hospital that doesn't.

In this chapter, we have not sought to develop any iron-clad specifics on these variations. Consultations with your current staff members will give you a clearer picture of this situation than you could ever hope to gain from a book.

Instead, we have concentrated on developing the general framework for an effective medical and/or surgical staff, leaving the specific "wrinkles" of the custom-fitting process to the discretion and judgement of each individual administrator.

The organizational framework is really the most important element in the development of an effective and efficient medical staff. The minor variations within the format merely serve to closely fit the abilities and personalities of the individual practitioners to the confines of the staff framework.

If this factor is kept in mind, permitting a limited amount of slack to exist in the system, most of the potential for friction among staff members, administration, and the hospital's governing board will be eliminated. Eliminating this friction is the largest single secret of efficient delivery of quality health care from your hospital to the community.

PART 2 — HOW TO MAINTAIN AN EFFECTIVE WORKING RELATIONSHIP WITH YOUR MEDICAL STAFF

One area of concern for many medical staffers, as they view their relationship with the hospital's administration, is the aloofness which many administrators seem to have in regard to the daily activities of the staff. While some individual physicians might prefer to be left alone to function with minimum administrative supervision, most physicians seem to prefer an administrator who is *involved* in the operational activities.

Essentially, this involvement most often takes the form of close communications with the medical staff on an informal basis. This informal approach, bridging the gap between the regularly scheduled formal staff meetings, often has a beneficial effect.

CASE IN POINT: IMPROVED COMMUNICATION HALTS HOSPITAL'S DANGEROUS MEDICAL STAFF EXODUS

A midwestern hospital had suffered, over a period of several years, from a major communications problem between the administrator and the medical staff—creating a climate that caused a substantial percentage of the staff to leave the hospital's service (or to consider doing so).

When a new administrator was appointed for the hospital, his first action was to make regular visits to the medical staff lounge. By making himself available for informal discussions, he effectively opened new avenues of communications between administration and the medical staff.

As a direct result of this single action, the trend of physician departures was halted. The overall morale of the medical staff markedly improved. As an added benefit, the medical staff was upgraded to have a full, required contingent needed to provide top grade hospital medical services. This improvement was accomplished within 18 months of the new administrator's arrival.

Getting Actively Involved

The preceding case example clearly illustrates the need for administrative *availability* in its relationship with the medical staff. There is no way that you can develop medical staff loyalty to your hospital if the lines of communication are not open.

While the formal medical staff meetings are often a good forum to discuss pertinent operational issues of hospital management, the formal nature of this setting rarely lends itself to the discussion of the small intangible factors which can have a major effect on staff morale.

As mentioned in Chapter 1, discussion and persuasion tend to be more effectively accomplished in the informal atmosphere. The relaxed "brain-storming" session can often yield surprisingly productive results. Ideas which can take the form of "Wouldn't it be interesting if we tried this method?" can prove to be a major source of administrative inspiration.

Be opening yourself up to these opportunities, you might be able to improve your own performance while at the same time improving hospital conditions to more accurately reflect the objectives and desires of your medical staff. There is probably no greater morale builder for the medical staff than to see one of their ideas being implemented by the hospital's administration.

Strengthening Hospital-Medical Staff Ties

When an administrator looks for ways to more closely tie the medical staff to the interests of the hospital, the tendency is to look for psychological, rather than tangible financial, anchors to motivate staff member behavior. Much to the annoyance of the administrator, this strategy rarely seems to work.

With an increased practice-management awareness within the medical profession, your administrative actions must be modified to meet this motivation head-on. Basically, you must look for ways to make a close alliance between doctor and hospital financially beneficial to the physician. If this brings added dividends to the hospital as well, your hospital's financial position will really be enhanced.

To fully understand how this general concept can be specifically developed to mutually benefit the hospital and participating physicians, let's take a look at some tested options at work.

(1) Shared Billing Systems

One major area of concern to the physician's practice-management plan is the area of accounts receivable. Considerable amounts of office staff time must often be devoted to the process of writing out and mailing bills to patients. The costs involved in this process can put a substantial dent in the gross revenues of the doctor's private practice.

One possible solution to this problem is to combine private-practice billing with the daily accounting activities of the hospital's business office. This can be most easily accomplished when a hospital's accounting practices are computerized. But this is not an absolute requirement for implementing this system.

In exchange for providing this service to the physicians, the hospital could receive minor renumeration from the participating physician. But this cost would inevitably represent a substantial savings to the doctor, providing an opportunity for expansion of practice capacity or reducing office staffing requirements. If the first possibility becomes an actuality, this could have a substantial positive impact on the hospital's service utilization picture.

In addition, this billing service could provide for better utilization of the Business Office staff, keeping productivity at a high level and preventing wasted time due to lack of available work.

CASE IN POINT: INNOVATIVE BILLING IDEA GENERATES OVER 15 PERCENT OF BUSINESS OFFICE'S OPERATING COSTS

One hospital in the western U.S. devised a system of billing private practice patients in cooperation with members of its medical staff. The agreement between the hospital and participating staff members stipulated that approximately 5 percent of the gross proceeds from such billing would be retained by the hospital as its renumeration for providing the service.

The net result of this program was a major cut in the physician's billing costs, approximately 50 percent. In addition, this added revenue helped to absorb over 15 percent of the Business Office's operating costs.

This major improvement in business methods had a substantial beneficial impact on both physician and hospital. With such benefits accruing from affiliation with the hospital, it is no surprise that this hospital has one of the highest physician retention rates in the country.

(2) Co-operative Purchasing Agreements

Another area of concern for private-practice physicians is the cost of office and medical supplies, plus general purpose medical instruments. Escalating costs are a concern for them as well as for hospitals.

One mutually beneficial possibility is to pool the purchases of private-practice physicians and the hospital together. By purchasing in larger quantities, some major monetary savings for both doctor and hospital can be realized.

**CASE IN POINT: CO-OP BUYING PLAN GENERATES ENCOURAGING
RESULTS FOR PHYSICIANS AND HOSPITAL**

One hospital in the southern U.S. developed a cooperative purchasing agreement with its physicians to buy supplies at quantity rates. This united buying strategy was particularly beneficial to the medical practitioner, reducing supply costs by over 30 percent on affected goods.

This method also proved beneficial to the hospital, permitting a 5 to 7 percent cut in its supply costs, thanks to the larger quantity rates.

The method used to implement this idea was to centralize all supply requisitions at the hospital's purchasing department. Each participating physician was provided with a standard form used by the hospital for this purpose. This standardization permitted the purchasing department to take on this additional responsibility without a decrease in departmental efficiency.

When these unified shipments were received, the orders for each physician were filled from the hospital's storeroom as per the original requisition and/or purchase order filed by the physician's office.

This method is particularly good if the doctors' offices are housed within the hospital. Supply transfers can be accomplished within the framework of normal hospital operations. Obviously, physicians with offices outside of the hospital would have some reduced efficiency due to the decentralized supply source. This loss of efficiency could potentially negate the financial benefits gained by the cooperative purchasing program.

SPECIAL LEGAL ADVISORY

Though this is usually considered, and treated as, a wholesale transaction between the hospital and the participating physician, a check with your attorney might be advisable to determine possible antitrust implications (if any).

Another Safeguard: It would be wise to advise participating physicians that they may be liable for direct payment of sales taxes on these purchases to their state treasury department. However, similar transactions, if conducted by individual physicians with out-of-state supply firms, would normally be exempt from such tax restrictions. Therefore, it's unlikely that this arrangement would represent any major legal problem.

Benefits: The Key to Physician Loyalty

Considering today's sociological climate, the rule of "money talks" is often the key to making solid professional relationships which can withstand the minor differences of opinion that will inevitably arise. In terms of developing productive working relationships with your medical staff, you must be on the alert for any opportunities to make your physicians more financially dependent upon your hospital. Each technique that provides a financial benefit for the practitioner will strengthen his or her alliance with the hospital.

This increased interdependence will also make your control of medical staff activities easier to carry out. Though staff members may not always agree with the programs which you and your board of trustees might wish to implement, their financial interests will prevent a major rebellion or reduction in overall morale. Weighing the benefits, as opposed to the negative factors, they will come to the conclusion that things could be worse.

Provided that your administrative planning doesn't become a virtual dictatorship, precluding medical staff input entirely, your relationship based on the beneficial aspects of your hospital's program can survive the minor problems that are a natural part of any human relations scenario. *

---

* See also ¶5001 *et seq.*, Prentice-Hall *Hospital Cost Management Service.*

How to avoid an adversary relationship with your board of trustees

THOUGH YOUR POSITION AS ADMINISTRATOR makes you, in effect, Commander-in-Chief of general hospital operations, the ultimate authority for hospital policies rests as the domain of your board of trustees. To meet your administrative objectives and implement plans, the support and concurrence of the Board are essential. If you fail to get their approval, the overall effectiveness of your position will be seriously compromised.

To meet this challenge, be prepared to "sell" your proposals to the board members, individually and as a group, to get the desired results. Your position, on a small scale, is similar to that of the President of the United States. He, too, must get Congressional approval to implement most of his plans.

The board members, serving in a voluntary capacity for the benefit of the hospital, are normally receptive to reasonable proposals forwarded by an administrator, provided that the administrator is willing to do his homework in preparing his presentations. This factor, more than any other, can determine your effectiveness in dealing with the hospital's board of trustees.

With primary responsibility to the community which they serve, members of the board continually scrutinize any proposals on this basis: "What is in the best interests of the community?" If your proposals are presented to directly address this question, chances of approval will greatly improve.

Composition of the Board

To insure maximum success in dealing with a hospital's board of trustees, a small amount of generalized background on the formation of hospital boards would be advantageous.

Generally, the composition of a hospital board tends to vary from community to community, depending on the societal make-up and the people available to serve on the board. As a rule, the number of board members ranges between 7 and 15.

Their selection is usually based on the background, knowledge, integrity, proven decisiveness and intelligence they have displayed in functions outside the realm of the hospital.

In an effort to best serve the community's interests, board membership usually reflects a microcosm of the social structure of the community. It is generally considered good policy to include members with special interests and skills, such as clergymen, bankers, contractors, editors, educators, and the like, to give the board a balanced view of the issues presented to it.

Some question has been raised regarding the appropriateness of including members of the medical profession on the governing board. Organizations such as the American Medical Association, the American College of Physicians, and the American College of Surgeons have officially gone on record supporting the concept of medical memberships on hospital governing boards. This membership, supporters claim, provides necessary background for the board to make intelligent decisions regarding medical matters. The opposition states that this function and input can be obtained equally well through consultation with the joint conference committee of the hospital's medical staff.

Whichever method is utilized, there is a clear need for medical knowledge in many of the decisions reached by the board of trustees. Hospitals that have decided against inclusion of a medical staff member of the governing board have made it a standing practice to invite the chief of staff to attend board meetings, in a non-voting capacity, to offer expert advice and counsel on matters involving medical procedures, equipment, etc.

By gaining this medical staff input, board members, otherwise unacquainted with the intricacies of medical science, can gain a greater understanding and appreciation of the various elements involved in the medical and surgical decision-making process. This knowledge is important to avoid decisions counterproductive to the objective of the medical administration of the hospital.

In a few of the larger hospitals, where the larger amount of board activity appears to warrant it, a full time chief executive officer is made a member of the hospital board. Operating under the title of President or Executive Vice President, this individual is found to be most useful where the extent of hospital investments, endowments, and other generalized holdings merits the full time attention of the hospital board.

If this system is utilized, the hospital board command structure would be altered somewhat, making the key volunteer member the Chairman of the Board. In any event, it is the volunteer portion of the board that wields the greatest amount of authority in the hospital setting.

Continuity vs. "New Blood": The Management Question

Tenure and transition in the setting of the hospital board are questions that, in some instances, can present some difficulty in the hospital management picture. The question of experience, as opposed to the need for new ideas, is one which can prove vexing. A single large turnover of board membership can prove counterproductive, at least in the short term, because it disrupts continuity of hospital policy. The need for a stable management policy is a vital public relations asset that can't be taken too lightly. This is a factor that encourages public confidence in any health care provider.

By the same token, if the hospital board has no noticeable changeover, this can lead to stagnation and can prove counterproductive in the pursuit of health care excellence. Another consideration is that some members, feeling that their tenure is "immortal", are likely to become unresponsive to the needs perceived by the community.

To answer the dual challenges of this problem, the conventional wisdom has been to rotate membership on a three-year term, with one-third of the board being changed annually. This allows two-thirds of the board to serve as a stabilizing continuity influence, with the one-third new membership serving as the source of new ideas from the community.

An effective argument could be made that this system can result in the loss of some effective board leaders with specialized expertise, a possible detriment to the efficient management of a hospital. In some instances, board members might be appointed to two consecutive three-year terms on the board. However, a one-year lapse between terms is advisable to prevent a proprietary attitude among board members.

Board members who retire from active duty in hospital governance should be encouraged to become the institution's "Good Will Ambassadors" to the community, promoting the hospital to improve the services it renders patients.

Continuing Education: A Vital Link

As periodic changes in the hospital's board membership occur, the need for continuing education of the Board becomes increasingly evident. New appointees may have some difficulty correlating their experiences outside the hospital environment with the problems that are faced in hospital management.

As administrator, it is your function to make sure that these new board members receive proper orientation in the elements of hospital management. The orientation process could include such items as the guided tour of the hospital facilities, detailed review of the various departmental processes, finances, and a host of other items which are involved in hospital management. This orientation procedure is an important safeguard for you because it tends to prevent new board members from unwittingly advocating procedures and policies which are obviously detrimental to the hospital's function.

In addition to your personal involvement in the orientation process, new and existing board members would benefit from some specific items of reading. Some of the suggested reading would be:

HEALTH IS A COMMUNITY AFFAIR, by the National Commission on
    Community Health Services (Harvard University Press, Cambridge,
    MA 1966)
TODAY'S HOSPITAL, by Raymond P. Sloan (Harper & Row, New York,
    1966)

HOSPITAL TRUSTEESHIP, by Dr. Charles U. Letourneau (Starling Publications, Chicago, 1958)

HOSPITAL POLICY DECISIONS—PROCESS AND ACTION by Arthur B. Moss, Wayne G. Broehl, Jr., Robert H. Guest, and John W. Hennessey, Jr. (G.P. Putnam's Sons, New York, 1966)

HANDBOOK FOR HOSPITAL TRUSTEES, by Dr. J.R. McGiboney (Hospital Publications, Inc., College Park, MD 1965)

Trustee, a monthly journal published by the American Hospital Association (considered MUST reading for the informed and effective hospital trustee)

In addition to reading these items, hospital board members should be encouraged to attend local, regional, and national hospital meetings to gain a further insight into national trends and developments in the field of hospital management. This added information will make your board members more effective in their task.

Basic Board Organizational Principles

In order to maintain the efficient operations of a hospital, its board must also operate according to standards conducive to meeting recognized management objectives. Depending on the business that the hospital board is required to conduct, the organization may be relatively simple or extremely complex. This is most often determined by the size of the hospital as well as the number of services it renders to the community.

To expedite the handling of hospital business, the hospital board will often be segmented into smaller working committees to review essential hospital business and make recommendations for final action by the complete Board. This committee structure provides an opportunity for members with specific expertise to serve in a review capacity for proposals brought for board considerations. If the proposals are obviously unworkable, the committee structure will provide a safety mechanism to prevent irresponsible actions from taking place.

Basically, the hospital board committee structure revolves around four essential entities. These are (1) the Executive Committee, (2) the Joint Conference Committee, (3) the Professional Committee, and (4) the Finance Committee. Other hospital board committees could be formed as business needs for the hospital dictate. Two examples of these additional committees would be Public Relations and the Building and Grounds committee.

Serving under commonly recognized bylaws adopted for the functioning of hospital boards, these committees tend to streamline the legislative process of hospital management. The committees provide close scrutiny of proposals without requiring the entire board to become involved in the research process that some programs might entail.

When the committees have reviewed proposals for their merits and ramifications in the management picture, they prepare a detailed report for presentation to the complete hospital governing board. After reviewing the condensed account of the committee's review, they can take final action on a reasonably intelligent basis.

To give us a more complete picture of the process, let's make a brief review of the functions of these four basic committees, serving as a brief refresher course on the subject.

(1) The Executive Committee

This committee, normally consisting of the president, secretary, treasurer, and the chairpersons of the other standing committees within the hospital, tends to serve as "the bottom of the funnel" for board committee functions. The executive committee provides the final review and evaluation for all other committee reports.

Authority for the executive committee is sweeping; in some cases it is equal to that of the entire governing board. This is particularly true in emergency situations where any delays might prove detrimental to the health and safety of patients and staff members alike.

Delegation of board tasks is another important facet of the executive committee's function. The executive committee is fully empowered to appoint temporary or ad hoc study committees to research specific areas of hospital management. This area is particularly important to the management picture because it permits the concentration of expertise among available board members to do the most effective job for the best interests of the hospital.

The executive committee, in short, plays a pivotal role in the formulation of hospital policy. As the center of power in the hospital board structure, it is this committee that could decide whether your ideas "live or die."

If you have done your homework and can "sell" this committee on the merits of your proposals, your chances of getting approval from the entire hospital governing board will improve drastically.

(2) The Joint Conference Committee

Earlier in this chapter, we discussed the vital necessity of maintaining close communications links between the hospital's governing board and the medical staff. The Joint Conference Committee serves as this communications link.

As you may recall from our detailed discussion of the joint conference committee which appeared in Chapter 3, the primary committee function is to serve in a liaison capacity between the medical staff and the hospital's governing authority, the combination of the administration and the hospital board.

Maintaining this committee as an effective, working entity within the governing structure should serve as reasonable assurance that governing board actions will not prove detrimental to the best interests of your hospital's patients or to the state of the medical art practices by your physicians and surgeons.

(3) The Professional Committee

In terms of the legal ramifications of hospital management, the Professional Committee probably holds the most sensitive role of any governing board committee. The delicate balancing act which is involved in the continuing operations of this committee makes the total legal responsibilities here formidable.

The professional committee, as an entity, holds the legal responsibility for maintaining the quality of hospital medical care. Because the committee is dominated by laymen, it can, on occasion, create a difficult question of diplomacy. While the governing board can never exercise direct control over how a physician treats a patient, court precedent *(Darling vs. Charleston Community Hospital*; Illinois Supreme Court, 1965) does clearly indicate that the legal responsibility for proper patient care is shared equally between the attending physician and the hospital in which treatment is given.

This clearly leaves the professional committee with the role of monitoring hospital staff activities to avoid, whenever possible, negligent actions which could prove detrimental to the health and safety of patients. Through the implementation of mutually acceptable bylaws and procedures, the professional committee can institute disciplinary actions against staff members to meet its legal obligations and to reduce the risks of litigatory actions against the hospital.

In addition to the monitoring function, this committee is also responsible for establishing and reviewing all hospital policies designed to maintain and enhance the quality of medical care.

Though the members of the professional committee will probably have greater expertise in the areas of finances, physical facilities and general administrative problems, their knowledge of medical administration should be sufficiently high to enable them to discharge their monitoring capacity effectively.

Clearly, the effective and efficient operations of the professional committee are dependent on the understanding and cooperative efforts of the governing board, medical staff, and administration. If this vital bond should ever break down, serious medical, legal, and administrative problems could soon overwhelm the best laid plans for your hospital's success.

(4) The Finance Committee

As the name implies, this committee is responsible for monitoring the monetary aspects of hospital operations. Working in close cooperation with the controller and administrator, it reviews the hospital budget and recommends policies designed to enhance institutional solvency.

Also included among committee duties is the review of financial statements and monitoring the on-going implementation of the hospital budget. By examining any budgetary variances which might occur, they can arrive at a consensus as to the need for policy changes during the term of the hospital budget. For example, if any hospital department has drastically departed from its projected budget (without substantial, unavoidable reasons provided for this occurrence), the finance committee could recommend specific cuts to bring the departmental budget back into line. These recommendations would, in turn, be implemented by the concurrence of the Administrator and Controller.

The checks and balances on the status of hospital finances provided by the committee offer a vital link in the total hospital administrative picture. The effective and knowledgeable functioning of the finance committee can serve as a valuable adjunct to the *team management concept* every hospital needs to achieve and maintain its success within a community.

Mutual Trust and Rapport: The Key Element

Your effectiveness as hospital administrator is clearly dependent on the relationship you develop with the governing authority. You can never afford to minimize the impact of a productive mutual trust between yourself and members of the hospital board.

In most cases, an administrator is selected because he is trusted by the majority of the governing board. The problem is narrowed down to maintaining this trust.

One of the first considerations in maintaining this necessary trust is to eliminate, whenever possible, the element of surprise in any proposals which you might present to the board. The worst method you could possibly adopt is to bring in a proposal "cold" without communicating its essence to chiefs of any departments affected or with a considerable number of the board members.

Laying the groundwork can be a tricky psychological balancing act. The best method to get this facet of the problem resolved is to inform board and staff members of any deliberations which you might be conducting. For example, if you are considering changes in the methods employed by the nursing staff, your best course of action would be to meet with the Director of Nursing in advance of making a final decision. By informing the director of the various factors which you are considering, you can not only keep the nursing staff informed, but can gain some valuable insights from them for your decision-making process.

In applying this principle to the board of trustees, you might want to call in a few committee chairpeople and other influential board members. There's a lot of truth in the unofficial business axiom that "Much persuasion is accomplished over a cup of coffee."

By using this initial unofficial approach, you can "warm up" the necessary people to the underlying concept of your proposal. When you have given them the chance to consider your ideas in a non-pressurized atmosphere, you will find them more receptive to proposals when they are formally presented.

The Formal Board Presentation

When you have laid the essential groundwork, by permitting your ideas to be in circulation for a month or two, you should be ready to make your formal presentation to the hospital's governing board.

What are the essential elements of an administrator's presentation? Clearly, doing your homework in advance is extremely important. You should have as many facts and figures as possible to serve as the background and rationale for your proposals. Board members will want to know two essentials on any proposals; (1) how the proposal will work, and (2) why you want the proposal implemented for your hospital.

This means that your presentation should include all pertinent information regarding the financial and health care impacts which you project for the proposal. You should inform the board honestly whether or not you can project that a proposed project will pay for itself, and, if so, in what projected time frame.

If a proposed project is not expected to be self-supporting, or incapable of returning the projected investment made in it, you must base your advocacy on the improvements in patient care environment or other pertinent factors. In any case, your proposal must be based on the *positive benefits* which the change will bring to the hospital.

When you get negative viewpoints from staff members to a proposal, you should honestly report these to your Board of Trustees. For example, a proposal for a change in medical care procedure may not get an enthusiastic endorsement from your medical staff. If, however, the change would result in a noticeable cost reduction for your hospital, you have a fairly good chance of having the Board approve the change, over the objections of the medical staff.

For this reason, your proposal presentation procedure may occasionally seem like a debate against yourself. But it serves the useful purpose of presenting the various items and views on the proposal, with emphasis from you on why the changes should be adopted. If you can honestly present both sides of the coin to the board, you will gain their respect and retain their trust. This will lower their resistance and make your management objectives easier to achieve.

Favoritism and "Conflict of Interest": The Administrative Crisis

The greatest danger to a productive relationship between an administrator and his board of trustees can come from the backgrounds which individual members can bring to their board duties. Since they represent various elements of the business and professional community, it seems unavoidable that, at some point, their outside interests will come into direct conflict with a hospital's business management. Any administrator who fails to recognize this does so at his own professional peril.

Here, again, we must take you back to the concept of completeness in your presentation. As an example, consider the possibility of purchasing malpractice liability insurance to protect the hospital. In shopping for this protection, you would undoubtedly get bids from a number of insurance companies.

The problems for your administration could begin if you had several insurance representatives on your board of trustees (not an entirely uncommon occurrence).

If you decided to choose one insurance carrier over the others for presentation and board approval, your choice of technique could leave you wide open for antagonism from some board members. If you present only the bid which you want the board to approve, you could be stepping into the proverbial hornet's nest. If the presented bid is from a member of the board, and another member is also an insurance representative, you could be accused of playing favorites with an individual board member.

This situation can degenerate quickly to make your relationship with the board a quagmire of dissension and ill will. If there is a suspicion that you have favored one board member over another, even on one occasion, you will be faced with skepticism and resistance on every proposal you present. Quickly your authority over hospital operations will erode, leading to a management crisis and chaos.

CASE IN POINT: ADMINISTRATIVE "FAVORITISM" SPARKED FINANCIAL CRISIS AT CENTRAL U.S. HOSPITAL

Consider the scenario which developed at a hospital in the central U.S. In 1977, this hospital showed a profit of $100,000. After a single miscalculation by the administrator (of the type mentioned above), board inflexibility set in.

In 1978, the hospital showed over $250,000 worth of red ink in their ledgers. Board resistance to administrative proposals turned the financial situation from a profitable one into a dangerously unstable one. In December, 1978, the administrator was relieved of his duties.

The clear solution to preventing this problem is to make sure that your presentation incorporates the following two elements:

(1) Present all bids and/or pertinent facts on any proposals presented to the board.
(2) Explain, in detail, the steps in your deliberation which lead to your final decision.

In going back to our example of the insurance policy, when you present all bids to the board, those board members who placed bids for consideration would abstain from voting (the conflict of interest question), and board action could proceed along its normal channels.

By opening up your deliberation process to board scrutiny, you can avoid ending up on the hot seat, having other board members coming to you asking for favors. In keeping all transactions on a strictly business basis, without even an appearance to the contrary, your integrity and authority with the governing board will not be diminished or destroyed.

CASE IN POINT: CONTRASTING POLICIES CREATE DIFFERING PROBLEMS FOR TWO HOSPITALS

For one western metropolitan hospital of approximately 1,200 beds, the acquisition of major supply items proved to be a major problem. Despite a sealed bid setup, a problem developed when a member of the hospital's board submitted a bid for consideration. Though the board member's bid was the lowest offered, it was rejected because of the possible conflict of interest considerations.

Because the lowest bid was rejected for other than product quality considerations, this hospital was canceled by several major insurance companies as an approved hospital. As a direct result of these insurance company actions, the hospital suffered a reduction in patient census (average) of over 15 percent.

By the same token, a 600-bed hospital in the Midwest had two members on the board who offered similar products for sale. When a bid was requested and a contract was awarded to one supplier, the other became quite angry and promptly canceled its standing contract for other supply items being furnished to the hospital. In addition, the angry board member resigned any further affiliations of any sort with the hospital.

Solution: The hospital sought a new source of supply for the canceled items and selected a new board member.

These two examples clearly illustrate the fine line which must be walked in these matters. In order to avoid these problems, some precautions might be in order. First, check with your most frequent third-party payers regarding their policy. If they have no objection to omitting potential bids from board members, you can avoid the public relations problems which this apparent insiders's advantage can create.

However, if insurance carriers (or your state regulations) require that bidding be open to all potential applicants, be certain that all parties are treated on an equal basis. This means that identical specifications data are provided to all bidders and no deadline extensions are permitted for any participants in the process.

This will eliminate any possible appearance of favoritism for any particular bidder. If these major considerations are met, there should be no relevant reason to block any possible bidders from entering into competition. This also assures that your hospital will gain the advantages offered by the most favorable pricing policies available.

CAUTIONARY NOTES ON CONFLICT OF INTEREST

The problem of dealing with hospital board members as suppliers can prove to be the proverbial "sticky wicket." Many hospital officials flatly refuse to do any monetary transactions with members of their Board because of the potential public relations problems which might ensue.

If there is any potential for questioning purchase policies, the best course of action would appear to be securing sealed bids from a variety of suppliers. If, under this system, the board member submitting a bid proves to be the best available, any questions regarding the propriety of the transaction will be effectively eliminated.

Likewise, possible problems with Medicare or any other third-party payers will be limited because their main concern is in effective cost containment—not in your source of supply.

The Administration-Board Relationship: Final Thoughts *

In rating hospital administrators for effectiveness, the clear winners will always be those individuals who have an amicable and business-like relationship with their governing boards. Though all interactions between the administrator and various elements of the hospital are important, none is more crucial to administrative success than the relationship with the governing board.

Without question, your effectiveness hinges on being able to get board concurrence for your plans and objectives. Maintaining a positive relationship here can easily be counted as 50 percent of the total challenge.

One hospital controller probably stated it best when he said: "Successful hospital management must be a total team effort. It's like a wheel with spokes. If one spoke is broken, the wheel wobbles. If two are broken, it wobbles even more. But if things deteriorate with the Board, that amounts to a broken axle. That brings the wagon to a halt."

Given the information in this chapter, you should be able to keep the "axle" solid and keep your hospital on the smooth road to success. *

---

* For more specifics, see ¶3101 *et seq.*, Prentice-Hall *Hospital Cost Management Service.*

The key service for hospital solvency

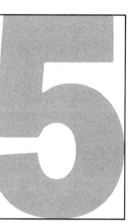

ONE OF THE KEY AREAS that can easily determine the financial success or failure of a hospital is the organization and operation of its Business Office. Under the generalized heading, Financial Services, this department handles the daily details of implementing a hospital's budget and internal financial controls. If any single portion of this vital apparatus goes into disarray, the financial results for the hospital involved could be catastrophic.

The financial services section is an extremely broad-based one, encompassing a considerable number of public contact elements of hospital business. Among the responsibilities here are personnel, admitting, credit and collections, insurance claims handling, communications, cashiers, internal control systems, payrolls, cost centers and budgets, central dispatch, and the mail and courier services.

Clearly, if it involves money in any way for the hospital, the broad range of financial services becomes involved. The objective of this chapter will be to dissect and analyze the functions of this vital hospital department, noting the signs of strength and weakness which must be observed to insure that "all systems are GO."

The Primary Functions

As the hub of the hospital's financial wheel, the business office extends its influence, regarding money matters, to almost every department in the hospital. As the accounting and analytical arm of the administrative process, it must maintain an adequate accounting system for all income, expenditures, and hospital assets.

If these records are sufficiently detailed, the chief of the business office, sometimes referred to as the Controller, can quickly ascertain areas of inadequacy or inefficiency, bringing them to the attention of the administrative office for action.

Another important function of the business office is the development, coordination, and control of the hospital's budget. (Due to the complexity of the subject, as well as its importance, we will devote a separate chapter to this area. See Chapter 6.)

In the area of controlling the budget, the business office maintains and develops purchase procedures and storeroom controls to assure that adequate supply levels are maintained while, at the same time, preventing the incidents of expensive and unnecessary duplication. This procedure should include a detailed periodic inventory of all supplies. This inventory would assure that business office records are current, as well as check that supplies are not subject to theft or other improper uses. By checking the levels of supplies used as opposed to the amounts ordered, comparing these figures to that of the inventory, the Controller can easily tell if every department has been keeping adequate records of their materials and supply usage.

As an allied function, the business office compiles pertinent patient and departmental statistics in conjunction with the medical records office. By maintaining detailed statistics, the business office, as well as the administrator, can keep a fairly close observation on the continuing functions of the various hospital departments and services.

Finally, and equally important, the business office prepares the financial reports, a crucial tool for an administrator and the governing board, serving as the basis for many of the decisions rendered. These financial reports bring, in condensed form, the needed information to make intelligent administrative decisions and safeguard the future financial health of the hospital.

Depending on the size of the hospital, these various functions may be held by a relatively few individuals or may be spread over a larger organizational entity. In any case, adequate supervision is required to insure that standards of competency and efficiency are maintained. This, in any event, is the responsibility of the business office and, more specifically, of the business manager or controller.

Qualifications at the Helm

Because of the diverse functions involved in the activities of the business office, the chief of this office must have a fairly large range of competency. While the controller should have equivalent qualifications to that of a Certified Public Accountant, this formal degree or certificate is not an absolute necessity. The important point is that sufficient business acumen, as that of a C.P.A., be present at the head of a hospital's financial services.

The business manager is directly responsible to the Administrator. The maintenance of this vital communications link, as well as those maintained with all other hospital departments, will determine the effectiveness with which he (or she) discharges the duties of the position.

The leadership factor is almost equally important to academic credentials in the performance of the job. Serving as a de facto second in command, the chief of financial services is a key link in the implementation process for management objectives.

This leadership will be particularly important in the budget formulation and monitoring process (the subject of Chapter 6, which we will examine in detail). Without this leadership, along with a considerable measure of authority over hospital activities, there is no way that a controller can do an effective job.

As one controller for a successful hospital stated: "If this office does not have the authorization and support from the administrator and the governing board to control hospital activities, they might as well lock the door to this office and not bother hiring a controller. Without the authority, the position has no value whatsoever to the hospital."

You and the Controller—A Constructive Bond

In effect, if not in actual fact, the most effective hospital management plan evolves around the team efforts of the administrator and the controller. The controller is your first line of defense against the financial problems which can beset a hospital.

Because the controller's office, with its staff, is best equipped to handle the flow of information from the various departments of the hospital, it is also the first to notice the development of problems. This line of defense is extremely important because a constant monitoring of a hospital's fiscal health is the *only way* it can be preserved.

The controller can, if you permit it, be an extremely valuable ally in your dealings with the hospital board. Because his "finger on the hospital pulse" is continuous in the course of his daily activities, he can explain to the board how the system is working. He can also explain *why* procedures are working, or not working, as the case may be.

For example, the hospital board might decide to implement a particular program for the hospital. But if, in actual practice, the program was not doing its intended function or proving detrimental to the hospital's financial picture, the controller could usually explain how the program was implemented, offering detailed reasons for its failure.

From your vantage point as the ultimate in-hospital authority, you may not have sufficient details to adequately explain the functions of every implemented program. Detail is the essence of a controller's job.

The real point of the working relationship between you and the controller is to give him adequate authority to do an effective job for you and the hospital. If the controller is doing his job, you can concentrate on the management theory and formulation of new ideas while he governs the implementation of administrative planning.

If this form of effective partnership is cultivated over a prolonged period, you should see major positive results in the general condition of your hospital.

FUNCTIONS WITHIN THE OFFICE

As mentioned at the start of this chapter, there are numerous functions which are allied to the basic function of Financial Services. In order to gain an adequate appreciation of the complexities of this operation, let's take an overview of the various functions performed.

The Admitting Office

The first contact between the hospital and the public it serves is, almost invariably, the Admitting Office. The speed and competency displayed here in handling the incoming patient's problems will often set the tone for how each individual views the services he (or she) receives.

For this reason, the public relations aspect of the office's function, often the least discussed, might be the most important single aspect of its service delivery. Often the manner in which patients' problems are handled will determine the total level of community support which the hospital will enjoy.

The emotions of people who come to the admitting office are often high. The tension factor, especially in emergency cases, is very high. Patients or their accompanying relatives are often "on edge," viewing the necessary admission procedures as an impediment to the hospital care they wish to have delivered.

A friendly and sympathetic attitude toward the patient's problem, as well as the related ones which involve the relatives, will often serve to bridge the time gap incurred by the necessary procedures.

One point of aggravation for patients, as well as contributing to hospital inefficiency, is the tendency to repeat similar questions at various stages of the admission process. Though obtaining information from the patient or relatives is a vital part of the total hospital care system, this can be streamlined in a mutually beneficial manner by providing an automatic method of disseminating pertinent data to the different hospital departments which will become involved in the patient's care.

The initial information gathering process should also be adapted, to some degree at least, to meet the needs and circumstances of the case involved. We've all seen the comedy sketches where an emergency patient is brought in for treatment, with a member of the hospital staff badgering the patient with useless questions. The most common illustration in this vein is the guy who comes in bleeding profusely. Then, he keeps getting asked (as he's bleeding dry), "What seems to be the problem?"

This is, of course, an exaggeration for the sake of comedy. But the situation does have its less ludicrous counterparts in many hospitals. The standing rule, at least in emergency cases, is to keep the quantities of trivia to a minimum. Just get enough information to get the initial treatment started.

Later, when the situation is less crisis-oriented, additional information can be obtained in a less stressful atmosphere. Additionally, if a long-standing file of patients is maintained (particularly if these records are computerized), the admitting office can cover the matters of medical records, credit history, and other items pertinent to the hospital stay by simply asking if the patient has been in your hospital before.

If the individual has been a patient in your hospital before, your admitting office can simply get the information from the computer's memory bank. This is just one example of a benefit of computerizing the Business Office, a subject we will discuss later in this chapter.

The fundamental goal of your Admitting Office should be to eliminate any physical or psychological impediments in the patient admission process to the largest extent possible.

The personnel of the admitting office, in order to meet management objectives, must maintain a demeanor which inspires confidence and assures those who give information that their personal affairs will not become matters of public scrutiny. This quality, though not necessarily acquired with age, is more often found in more mature employees.

This sympathetic quality should be teamed up with a keen perception of character types and the likely ability of the patient to pay his obligations to the hospital. Some sources have argued that the older, more mature employee might prove to be overly sympathetic to patients in this regard, more inclined to offer the benefit of the doubt in financial arrangements.

Admitting Office Policy Requirements

In order to adequately and uniformly serve the public, the admitting office must set up and maintain a solid set of standards for maintaining the Office as well as procedures for admission. Though these requirements might vary slightly according to the individual needs of the hospital, certain common sense elements must be maintained for proper Office operations.

These policy elements should include:

(1) Continuous 24-hour-a-day, 7-days-a-week coverage of the admitting office.
(2) Preventing delays of any emergency patients in order to get information.
(3) Developing and maintaining a rotating system of staff doctors to render care for patients who have no physician.
(4) Providing for examination by a physician of any patient who is refused admission and having reasons for this action explained by the examining physician or the hospital administration.
(5) Selection and adoption for use of pre-admission forms.
(6) Arranging for the supply of doctors' offices.
(7) Getting a signature, on the required form, from any patient who decides to leave the hospital against his doctor's advice.
(8) Explaining billing system to patients.
(9) Depositing and safeguarding of patients' valuables in the hospital safe.
(10) Maintenance of appropriate hospital records.

The preceding ten elements of admitting office policy are generally recognized to serve the basic requirements for efficient service to the public.

Key $ and Timesaver

An excellent method to cut down on admitting office paper work (and overcome departmental objections to carbon copies that might smudge) would be to photocopy admission information to be sent to departments requiring it. This would eliminate the need for numerous originals prepared by the admitting office staff.

While this may not be the best possible alternative to solving the problem, it does offer several major advantages. First, it is quite inexpensive to set up. In many cases, this merely means an additional use for existing office equipment. Second, the simplified nature of the process assures that it can be quickly picked up by new employees, a very important consideration in a hospital where clerical staff turnover is particularly high.

The Accounting Department

Within the financial "heart" of every hospital, this essential subdivision serves as the "pacemaker" which keeps the monetary flow at the most even rate possible. The accounting department serves the vital function of dealing with the extensive paper work that's commonly required to get the money in.

Dealing with the large variety of forms required to satisfy the needs of government agencies and the multitude of insurance carriers that cover hospitalization expenses for their subscribers can be a formidable task. While many insurance companies, for example, have helped by allowing standardized claim forms for requesting payment, the workload for even the small to medium-size hospital can prove quite large.

This workload, coupled with that provided by the private billing to patients for services not covered by insurance carriers, becomes so large as to represent a nightmare for the efficiency-conscious administrator. Although some successful efforts have been made to consolidate billing procedures, the barest minimum that must be accomplished can represent a considerable expense in terms of work hours utilized.

This influx of paper work has been a major contributor to the advance of computerization in hospital business offices across the country. This major time and labor-saving development, first initiated during the mid-1960's, has grown to become a major factor in hospital business management today.

Though the list of computerized hospitals continues to grow, there remains a major problem for those that do not have, due to financial constraints or other reasons, the computer capability. For them the term "business as usual" can have an ominous connotation.

To help in coping with this major source of problems, there are several techniques which can be utilized to effectively cut the amount of time required to handle the billing process. Let's briefly review a few of these ideas, possibly showing you how to implement them into your hospital's game plan.

(1) "Continuous" Forms

One major helpful innovation initiated by the form printing industry has been the development of the "continuous" form format. This method sets up the printed forms into a roll, very much like paper toweling, with perforations between each form to permit easy separation.

The most efficient layout for this type of operation would place the box of continuous forms at the back of the typewriter. This permits the insertion of the forms directly from the box into the typewriter. The single insertion to start the process, lining up the form for straight typing, is the only time the typist needs to perform this function for each session of bill or form preparation.

At the left of the typewriter, an incoming basket can contain the accounting records for those that will require billing. Removal from this basket to easy viewing range is the first step in the process. When the necessary information is transposed from the accounting record to the invoice, this record can then be placed in an "Out" basket located to the right of the typewriter.

With only a minimum of advance planning, remembering to remove all required records from the files, your office typist can prepare most, if not all, of the hospital's monthly invoices without wasted motion or movement from her position at the typewriter.

To re-cap this idea, here is a small illustration of the layout.

"IN" Basket Here	Box of Forms Here	"OUT" Basket Here
		Stack of Completed Forms Here
Record Viewing Area Here	Typewriter Here	

The key to making this idea work is the nature of the forms used. The increased efficiency is provided by the fact that, as each form is completed, the invoice is torn off at the perforation, ready to be placed into the mailing envelope. In advancing the form to be ready for removal, the typist automatically readies the next form for typing.

To illustrate the benefits of this idea, let's consider the results presented in the following case study of this system in action.

CASE IN POINT: CHANGE IN FORMS CUTS OVER 20 PERCENT OF BILL PREPARATION TIME

When the representative of a major printing firm visited the business office of one midwestern hospital, he discovered that the billing process was woefully inefficient. Many more motions than required were being performed by members of the hospital's typing pool.

After studying the situation, he recommended that the invoicing system be converted to the "continuous" form styling. For a minimum added cost, the amount of time for billing could be cut substantially (according to the representative).

The hospital bought the program, considering it for a short-term trial. The results after the first month were encouraging, an average 10 percent cut in the invoice preparation time. After the staff became accustomed to the new system, the results were even better. Within three months, the new system had shaved off over 20 percent of this crucial time-consumer.

Sold on the notion of this system, the hospital has begun to convert as many of its business forms as possible to the new system. The new idea, according to the hospital's controller, is expected to improve total productivity by a minimum 15 percent when fully implemented.

The real test of this system comes in terms of total cost effectiveness. The overall cost of this type of system runs approximately 8 to 12 percent above what is charged for standard individual forms. While many small local print shops may not have the equipment to provide this type of service, several major nationwide printing companies offer good prices and excellent service to get your business office started on the program.

Your best source of information would be a local company representative. If they are not listed under company headings in your phone directory, ask local businessmen or your local Chamber of commerce. Most of these people have been contacted by large printing company representatives at one time or another. They could probably give you the names and phone numbers of the people you wish to contact.

(2) "Semi-computer" Technology

Another possible solution, though a slightly more costly one, is to enter the computer utilization area at the ladder's bottom rung. Thanks to modern electronic wizardry, traditional typewriters are gradually giving way to a new breed. This hybrid is a mixture of the usual typewriter and limited computer function.

By combining the use of a Video Display Terminal with an interconnected printer, this "semi-computer" offers *some* of the advantages of computerization without the monumental cash outlay. At the time of this writing, the cost for the total system was in the $2,000 to $3,000 price range.

The Video Display Terminal offers several advantages over traditional typebar on paper methods used in the past. For example, typists' errors are not registered on paper, sometimes forcing the scrapping of entire forms. This facet alone, in some offices, represents a 3 to 5 percent savings in paper costs.

Second, some units can be programmed, like a computer, with the names of hospital accounts. With the touch of a single button, the name and address of the next account are automatically typed at the top of the account form layout on the display screen.

Third, when the form preparation is complete, all copies which must be acquired will be of original quality without the usual complaint of illegibility often attributed to carbon copies or the products of carbonless paper forms.

Most significantly, the step to Video Display Terminals will not be counter-productive if your hospital ultimately decides to go for total computerization. These same units, essentially small self-contained computers, can be adapted into a total hospital system.

A restricted version of this type of system (minus the display screen) is offered by the newest and most sophisticated electronic typewriters. Costing in the neighborhood of $1,000, these units have limited "memory" capabilities for facts. Units priced at the top range of the electronic typewriter spectrum have memory capacity for a full page of typescript, offering the advantage of "original" copies of forms with the touch of a single button on the unit.

Combining Ideas for Greater Payoffs

The two preceding ideas, particularly as they apply to the electronic typewriter, have produced some fairly substantial efficiency payoffs when implemented. By using the "continuous" forms with the sophisticated typewriters (using the one copy per typing form setup), the efficiency of the operation has been enhanced even further.

When the typing of one copy has been completed, the typist merely advances the form to the next copy by using the automatic return button. Then, with the pressing of another button, the second copy of the material is made. During this interim, the typist can be packing the "original" copy into the mailing envelope and reaching for the next account to be processed.

The results of this combination have proven favorable to the efficiency goal. To assess the results, let's look at a hospital that implemented the plan.

CASE IN POINT: COMBINATION PLANNING REAPS ADDED BENEFITS FOR EASTERN HOSPITAL

The essence of one eastern hospital's problem rested with the slow processing of accounts in their business office. Analysis revealed a considerable amount of wasted effort and time was involved in the work routine.

For example, each account billing was either photocopied or carbon copies were provided in the typing procedure. By either method, much time was involved in getting the work done.

Because the hospital's financial base did not permit the conversion to computers, the administrator decided to explore the possibility of using new electronic typewriters (with memory capacities) to help speed up the office production. After first renting a few units for a month or two (to assess the impact of the idea), the decision was made to proceed.

Using conventional equipment, this hospital would have been forced to spend an additional $17,000+ in the first year alone to get adequate productivity. With the investment of approximately $9,000 in equipment, the necessary production was achieved in the hospital's business office. The administration's initial plans to hire two additional typists were shelved.

Counting the investment required, the hospital's first year savings were in excess of $8,000. With future wage escalations considered, the elimination of staff additions here would save over $85,000 in a five-year period (after the first year's tally is completed).

Though some cases may be even more extreme than the one cited here, this clearly illustrates the wisdom of making an initial investment, though seemingly high, to reap future cost containment benefits. The long-term benefits of this program to the eastern hospital were magnified because enhanced efficiency ultimately opened the door to expanded duties for the business office, helping to bring added revenue for the hospital. But none of this would have been possible if this hospital's administration had not possessed the foresight to make the innovative plunge into modern electronic procedures.

Take some time now to consider the benefits which the new electronic "word processor" technology could reap for your hospital. You may find that your business office may be only scratching the surface of its ultimate performance potential under current conditions.

The Paper Traffic Center

Because of the complexity of hospital business, the area of financial services is often pressed into being a clearing house for most of the information pertaining to hospital business. The paper work that is generated by every revenue producing department is funneled into the hospital's business office. This pile of paper represents a problem that, if not properly handled, could become an organizational crisis.

If you consider the added load of paper required to record hospital expenditures, the scenario for a potential nightmare could easily be developed. For this reason, efficiency demands that the various subdivisions of function be firmly delineated in the office. Each specific area, from payroll to communications and central dispatch, must have a designated individual responsible for its smooth and efficient operations. If you lump together too many responsibilities on one person, none of the tasks will be accomplished to meet satisfactory standards of excellence.

While it's obvious that most hospitals would not need a full-time employee for each specific function, the consolidation of similar functions under one person's jurisdiction does seem to offer beneficial results. As an example, one individual might be responsibile for inpatient and outpatient billing, with the maintenance of credit account records as a related responsibility. Another individual might be responsible for the paper work of insurance company and government claim forms, the two being somewhat similar in nature. A third person could be assigned the internal communications detail, with the mail and courier services as an adjunct to the main duties.

The main idea is to develop proficiency in a general area of hospital operations. If one employee is required to spend a small portion of her day with payroll duties, another small portion with insurance and government claim forms, and yet a third small portion with patient billings, she whould have great difficulty developing sufficient familiarity with any of the functions to permit swift and efficient completion of the assigned tasks.

By keeping specific employee assignments to one general area, much of this potential confusion and reduced efficiency can be avoided. Centralization of function is the key element to enhancing the efficiency of any hospital's business office.

The Payroll Function

As the largest single expenditure in the management of any hospital, effective procedures for the monitoring and control of staff payroll functions are essential elements in maintaining the institution's financial health. Though there may be some psychological differences involved in dealing with various elements of the hospital's staff, depending on their education and status, the basic items involved in payroll monitoring must be applicable to all hospital employees.

The customary method used for monitoring employee time has generally been the time card/time clock combination. While this might present the possibility of cheating (someone punching in a fellow employee who isn't present), the increased efficiency of this system for the payroll clerk is generally recognized as negating potential drawbacks.

In the cases of professional staff members who might take offense at being treated like "common" employees, a logbook arrangement is sometimes substituted for the time card. The professional staffer simply signs in, including the time of arrival. He (or she) follows the same procedure before leaving the hospital at the end of each day.

The greatest single problem in payroll preparation is presented by the rules and regulations of the Internal Revenue Service and the various state treasuries that demand deductions from employee paychecks. The amount of paper work and record-keeping involved in meeting these requirements will often play a major role in determining the length of employee pay periods. The efficiency of your hospital's bookkeeping services could become strained to the limit if paydays come at too frequent intervals.

Because pay period lengths do play such an integral role in bookkeeping efficiency, this might be a good place to begin checking for problems if your current efficiency levels here are not up to par. In an effort to enhance employer-employee relations, some businesses attempt to issue paychecks at weekly intervals. If this is your case, you may be placing too great a drain on your available equipment and manpower to effectively and efficiently accomplish your hospital's bookkeeping functions.

The clear solution to this problem is to expand the length of your pay periods to ease the strain. This option is far less costly to the hospital than to purchase additional equipment or increase staffing to facilitate the increased workload. Though this may present a temporary problem for your employees, the adjustment can be accomplished within a reasonable period of time.

If your hospital employees are unionized (with the pay period arrangement as part of the contract), ask to have this matter as a topic of negotiation. By emphasizing the long-term best interests of the hospital's operation, with statistical analysis to back up your statements, you should have very little problems in gaining this needed accommodation.

To maintain an effective system, four items are generally recognized to be of prime importance to the efficient operations of payroll procedures. To consolidate the discussion, here, in capsule form, are the four items.

(1) Sample charts regarding salaries and hourly wages should be established for all employees of the hospital.
(2) Develop standardized policies regarding all overtime work, including pay rate and minimum hours before accelerated pay rates are put into effect.

(3) Method of payment. For efficiency reasons and ease of monitoring finances, payment by check is the best alternative.

(4) Modify all peripheral elements of the system to meet the needs of your individual hospital. Because each hospital is different in some small way, no single system can be instituted to suit every hospital.

The "bottom line" to all of this is to adapt your available ideas and resources to prevailing conditions. The payroll function, like every other aspect of your hospital's daily activities, must be sufficiently flexible to meet its goals as efficiently and economically as possible.

Accounting and The Third-Party Payment Process

As the source for most hospital revenue in today's economy, the accounting section's relations with various third-party payers—most significantly, the insurance companies—has assumed a critical importance. If the communications efficiency in this sector ever breaks down, dire financial problems for the hospital will usually result.

Considering the major reliance on computerization by major insurance carriers, along with an allied increase in the variety and complexity of telecommunication technology, the newest development has been to connect the computers of the billing party (in this case, the hospital) directly with the computers of the payer. This development has resulted in major time reductions in claim processing and has reduced the potential cash flow problems for participating hospitals.

How can you determine if your hospital can gain the maximum advantage from this system? To answer this question, review the items on the following checklist to determine economic feasibility.

CHECKLIST FOR "DIRECT LINE" COMPUTER USE

(1) Are your hospital's accounting functions currently being managed by computer?

(2) If so, is the computer equipped to provide direct access to telephone communications with the unit and a compatible unit on the outside?

(3) Are the insurance companies which currently provide over 50 percent of benefit revenue for your hospital equipped with compatible hook-ups to provide direct line communications?

(4) Can your current accounting department staff, with minimal additional training, adapt to the new operating system?

(5) Will a major renovation of Accounting Department facilities be required to accomplish this change of operational modes?

Checklist Results Reviewed

In a quick review of your results, "Yes" answers to Questions 1 and 2 are the most important considerations. This represents the core of any direct line computer billing system to insurance companies and would be non-functional without them.

Question 3 reflects on the cost effectiveness of such an innovative approach. If only a very small portion of your hospital's insurance paperwork were handled through this route, the cost effectivenss would be questionable—particularly if your current answer to Question 2 was negative. In order to fully justify the investment, a substantial percentage—preferably 50 percent or more—of your insurance revenue claims should qualify for this system.

Question 4, covering personnel qualifications to handle this system, represents a potential "thorn in the bed of roses" for this system. If substantial training would be required to retain current personnel for operating the system, these costs must be figured into your analysis.

The possibility of replacing current employees with people already qualified to handle the system could place a hospital in some very murky legal waters. Union agreements might require you to retain these employees in some other capacity within the hospital, though a "No Pay Reduction" clause might be in the agreement.

Watch This: This type of situation could thoroughly sabotage any cost savings which might be enjoyed by such a complete computer conversion. The only remaining benefit would be faster cash flow from insurance companies due to enhanced communications.

Question 5 addresses the serious question involving the hidden cost factor in any major operational change. While most of us would easily recognize the direct capital outlay for equipment changes, modifications of the existing physical characteristics of facilities can represent a major cost.

As an example, an office might be perfectly adequate to handle standardized equipment modes. However, when specialized equipment enters the picture, current space might prove woefully inadequate. If this factor is not taken into account in the initial planning stage, administrative planning can prove faulty.

Major equipment outlay commitments, taken without consideration of this factor, can put a severe strain on the hospital's budget. Literally caught "between a boulder and a hard place," the choices boil down to leaving the equipment unutilized—definitely a waste of money—or putting more money into the project by financing the facility renovation to accommodate the equipment.

Advance planning prevents this problem. Space is the hidden quantity which can effectively decide whether major computer conversion will ultimately prove to be financially viable for your hospital.

Special Problems of Credit and Collections

Because not all hospital fees are collected through insurance claims, we would be remiss in not making mention of another facet which could represent difficulty in the cash flow process—direct billing of the patient.

Aside from the basic mechanics of the operation, which we covered earlier in this chapter, the problem of nonpayment is probably of the greatest concern. The central issue in this area is to effectively differentiate between those individuals who are having financial difficulty and those who can be classified as chronic deadbeats.

While it is virtually impossible to create a completely airtight system to avoid being burned, there are acceptable techniques to avoid the bulk of potential problems. Some hospitals utilize a deposit system to prevent or reduce the incidence of delinquent accounts.

The deposit system requires a minimal deposit of money with the hospital, stipulating amounts varying from twenty-five to one hundred dollars, payable at admission, to be placed against the hospital's total bill. Though this system does appear to create some major public relations problems for the hospital, this can be minimized if the application is uniform with all patients.

Most hospitals will not go this route, opting instead to create firm financial arrangements for any amounts due. Uninsured amounts are often arranged for financing by a nearby bank.

This system offers several distinct advantages to the hospital. First, the hospital gets its money almost immediately. Accounting problems are minimized because no balances need to be carried over from month to month.

Second, if collection problems ensue, the hospital does not play the role of the "heavy," having to press for payment. The hospital's image remains unpolluted by such peripheral problems, thereby retaining its image as healer and health care provider for the community it serves.

The largest single benefit could likely be the effective reduction of interest charges that could be levied against the hospital when cash flow problems enter the picture. If a hospital needs to borrow money to gain essential operating capital, this can represent large dollar amounts. Double-digit interest rates, so prevalent at the time of this writing, merely serve to magnify the problem and multiply the benefits when this can be avoided.

This interest charge problem has two facets which can conspire to create major problems for any hospital unfortunate enough to confront them. First, if a major portion of a hospital's operating funds come from the bank loan source, the amount of operating capital is reduced by the amount of the interest. In addition, monthly installments to be repaid to the lender tend to make the financial management picture murky—at best.

The second facet is that the problem tends to be self-perpetuating. If a hospital has dug a hole for itself financially, it becomes increasingly difficult to get out of the position.

Prevention is the key. By transferring the financing obligation from hospital to patient, the major part of this crisis can be avoided completely. This puts your hospital in a much improved position to deal with the other financial problems which seem to be an inevitable part of management planning during these chaotic economic times.

The Business Office: Other Functions

Because this book will set aside specific chapters to offer more detailed discussion on some functions directly affected by business office policy and activity, we will offer only the briefest mention of them here, permitting you to make the interconnection between the various functions.

Other functions coming under the jurisdiction of the business office would include the Hospital Budget, Purchasing and Storeroom Controls, and the Personnel Department. In fact, virtually all hospital departments come, at one point or another, into the jurisdictional sphere of the business office's function. If it involves money, the business office has jurisdiction.

Some Concluding Thoughts

Throughout this chapter, our emphasis has been on developing an efficient operation pattern for your hospital's business office. Because it plays such a central role in the financial health of your hospital, the functions here *must* be at their finest. Any noticeable breakdowns in operational procedures here will have a ripple effect throughout the entire hospital, tending to distort all aspects of management and operations.

As stated in the early part of this chapter, this is the hub which permits the hospital's financial wheel to turn efficiently. Efficient equipment and modified procedures can go a long way in maintaining the optimum operations of this department.

But the most important part of the business office's success comes from the quality of its staff. In hiring employees who are dedicated to excellence, here, as in all other hospital departments, you can assure the best possible performance. No amount of procedural tinkering can make up for a lack of staff performance.

This, then, becomes your primary consideration. If you hire the right people for the business office staff, you can be reasonably assured of gaining the maximum benefits of enhanced management ideas for your hospital's future. *

---

* See also ¶3201 *et seq.,* Prentice-Hall *Hospital Cost Management Service.*

How to plan an effective hospital budget

PLANNING AND IMPLEMENTING THE HOSPITAL BUDGET is the cornerstone of any successful hospital management program. Serving as the guidebook for annual hospital operations, the budget is the only reliable vehicle for judging the success or failure of a management plan.

Without a budget, a hospital could be compared to a boat lacking propulsion and steering. Adrift in the "Sea of Ambiguity," no hospital administration can make intelligent management decisions. The essentials of the hospital budget pinpoint the current financial position of the institution, and outline where it is projected to go during the term of the budget.

Over a period of several months, during the developmental phases of the budget, every department becomes involved in the evolution of the final product. On the basis of departmental projections, along with other important factors to be discussed in this chapter, the hospital's controller can make a fairly accurate projection of the revenue requirements for the coming year.

When all of the various budget elements are compiled, the difficult management decisions regarding room rates and fees for the different hospital services can be made. Without a budget to serve as background for these decisions, administrative and board decisions would amount to "shooting blind," attempting to hit the target without knowing its location.

The Departmental Budget: The First Step

The initial step in the budgetary process begins at the department level. Each hospital department must, according to the average figures of the patient census (a budgeting factor to be discussed later), develop generalized cost projections for operating the department's activities.

To be an effective management tool, each departmental budget must include five essential sections. These would be:

    (1) Salaries of staff.
    (2) Cost of supplies.

 (3) Projected replacement of equipment.
 (4) Projected energy expenditures.
 (5) Miscellaneous (a contingency fund).

When the totals for these five budgetary elements are brought together and compared with the projected revenue which the department is expected to produce, the overall profitability of departmental operations can be determined.

 Though many hospitals are technically non-profit institutions, a favorable balance for each revenue-producing hospital department's income statement should be considered an essential part of the management program. Without it, the funds for capital outlay expenditures could be in short supply.

 To decipher the departmental budget a bit further, let's take a brief, but closer, look at the five elements involved.

(1) Salaries of Staff

 As the single largest factor in the departmental budget, staff salaries have a significant effect on the total profit picture of a hospital. Across the board, wages and salaries account for 50 to 60 percent of the total expenses of hospital management.

 This fact makes it imperative that each department chief review and closely scrutinize the staffing needs for his department. Though staffing requirements vary according to the nature of departmental activity, there must be some correlation between the department's workload and its level of staffing. If staff members have time to "view the scenery" or indulge in other nonproductive pursuits, this would indicate an overstaffing situation that is detrimental to the department's financial picture.

 As a counterpoint to this, hospital management should make every effort to provide adequate activity levels to keep minimum staffing occupied. In most hospitals, if this is not achieved, management is not aggressively searching for sufficient means of staff utilization. (This subject will be discussed in further detail in Chapter 21.)

 If this low activity situation becomes chronic, serious consideration must be given to eliminating the department completely. Except for the vital cornerstone departments of the hospital, this can often be done without major impact on the quality of care being delivered.

 One method to achieve this maximum utilization goal is to consider consolidation of services with nearby hospitals. For example, if your laundry is underused, you might want to consider taking in the laundry of a nearby hospital to augment the service load generated by your own facility. Another option is to close your laundry and farm out the work to another hospital.

 Either of these options would involve reasonably close cooperation between your office and the administration at another hospital. Maintaining efficiency with this type of arrangement could prove a stumbling block because it requires coordination between two separate management entities.

 Minimizing this problem requires that you select a hospital whose management philosophy and methods closely mirror your own. Also to be considered is the distance between the two cooperating hospitals. With energy costs being an increasing factor, the price tag for transporting materials between two hospitals could wipe out any cost savings you might receive from the move to service consolidation.

Whatever methods you might ultimately choose to implement, the bottom line consideration is that you receive enough revenue to justify the salaries paid out. You must get your dollar's worth of services rendered for every dollar paid out. If you don't, your chances for financial difficulties, particularly during periods of high inflation, will markedly increase.

(2) Cost of Supplies

Another major factor in the cost of health care delivery is the price tag for hospital supplies. Inflation has caused a marked increase in the percentage of the total hospital budget which is devoted to supply acquisition.

A CASE IN POINT: GROUP BUYING PLAN BRINGS THREE-DOLLAR CUT IN "PER PATIENT" COSTS FOR MICHIGAN HOSPITAL

One Michigan hospital conducted an "Inflation Survey" of the twelve most frequently used supply items on their premises. For a one-year period, the *average* inflation rate for the twelve items was an astronomical 56 percent.

Though the results of this 1979 survey were somewhat discouraging, the results could have been even worse. As the hospital's controller explained, their participation in a group buying program through a hospital association has resulted in an average saving of approximately $3.00 per patient in supply costs.

With a high inflation rate imposing itself on the hospital care marketplace, this factor must be included in any figures which are compiled for a hospital budget. If this is not taken into account, almost any budget could become a shambles before the ink dries on the printed sheet.

Every department chief, in determining the needs for his (or her) department, should carefully examine the cost escalation factors which have historically been imposed on the department's operations. A review of the preceding three to five years should give a fairly accurate perspective on the general direction of costs per patient. This, combined with a moderately accurate projection of the patient workload to be imposed on departmental activities, should give a clear picture of supply costs for the next annual departmental budget.

SPECIAL NOTE ON CONSULTATION:

While our recommendation does appear to grant some considerable autonomy for an individual department head, the need for direct consultation between department chiefs and the purchasing department is quite evident. The important thing to remember is that each department chief has a solid knowledge of costs for his area. If this cost knowledge is not present, there is little hope that an effective and meaningful departmental budget can be formulated.

If detailed explanations are offered for each budget item, most reasonable governing boards will agree to the budgets recommended. Each item should be accounted for in the detailed explanation. For example, a lab may be averaging 600 blood tests per month. This detail should be included, plus the current price and projected increase in the cost of needles and syringes.

If your presentation is detailed to this degree, no review panel could possibly reject the budgetary recommendations. The increases, particularly in this area, could be blamed on "unavoidable inflationary factors."

Here, as in every other facet of hospital management, the key word is *communications.* Keeping the people involved thoroughly informed as to the direction and intent of your administrative actions will help to lubricate the gears of the management mechanism.

(3) Projected Replacement of Equipment

Though this area could be placed under the heading of the Capital Outlay Budget, those items of equipment which are projected to require replacement during the term of the budget under consideration should be included in the annual departmental budget.

Under the heading of the Capital Outlay Budget, the long-term objectives and projections for equipment replacement are generally included. Due to the large price tag associated with many items of hospital equipment, this long-range planning is essential to be sure that the necessary financial assets are available to get the job done.

For this reason, department chiefs must classify departmental equipment according to expected useful life and determine when replacement due to wear or obsolescence will be required. Those items that are projected to be replaced during the coming year are placed in the annual departmental budget. The remaining equipment acquisition plans are placed on a long-term projection list which is maintained to facilitate administrative planning.

The long-term aspects of capital outlay expenditures for equipment are never really completed. It's an ongoing planning process between the department chiefs, the administration, and the governing board of the hospital. The major difficulty in this area lies in the rapid progress made in medical science and technology. New technology can often render hospital equipment obsolete only a year or two after it is acquired.

Another factor in the equipment acquisition and replacement question surrounds the variety and expansion of hospital services being offered to the community. Though the general equipping of a hospital is relatively standardized, some problems could be generated when new specialities and/or services are offered.

Generally, the best policy in this area is to make equipment purchases after you receive a firm commitment from a specialist to practice in your hospital. Because general hospital equipment is relatively standardized, as mentioned earlier, the hospital's budgetary outlay should be limited to a small amount of specialized instruments.

For example, to recruit a gynecologist for your hospital, you would have to assure this doctor that your hospital would provide the few gynecological surgery instruments that are specifically designed for his (or her) specialty. Aside from those few specialized items, the other items involved in the surgical procedures would be similar to those used by general surgeons.

The only exception to this pattern would be if your hospital's physical plant were so seriously deficient as to discourage new doctors from coming to your hospital on these grounds. If this happens, it reflects a serious gap in administrative planning and a life or death crisis for the survival of a hospital.

Your only recourse in this situation would be to engage in long-term financial planning to defray the costs of immediate structural improvements to meet the standards set by the modern medical profession. This type of expenditure would definitely be classified under the heading of the Capital Outlay Budget. Later in this chapter, we will show how this type of recovery procedure can be instituted for the "terminally ill" hospital.

(4) Projected Energy Expenditures

Though this factor is usually computed on a hospital-wide basis, it should nonetheless be considered in departmental activity planning. When you consider that prices for petroleum resources have skyrocketed by more than 500 percent particularly as they apply to heating and electrical generation, in the period between 1973 and 1980, there is no way to ignore the implications of these facts on the hospital management picture.

Department chiefs can, with a little analytical thought, consider the implications of their energy usage. Considering the costs involved, emphasis on efficiency and energy conservation methods would go a long way toward enhancing the overall profitability of the department and the entire hospital.

As grim as the current energy cost figures might be, even the most conservative energy resources analysts predict that *energy costs will double* between the years 1980 and 2000. International turmoil, particularly affecting the prime petroleum-producing regions, could substantially escalate this inflationary pressure.

The fact makes the "energy consumed vs. productive labor accomplished" question of extreme importance to the future management philosophy of hospital health care delivery. If you add the public pressures for cost containment to this picture, you can easily envision a serious crisis on the national health care horizon.

The only effective way to minimize the effects of this problem is to begin planning *now*, on the departmental level, to address the serious question of energy costs and conservation.

(5) Miscellaneous (a Contingency Fund)

At some point in every management plan, there must be a safety valve provided to meet the unexpected events which can ruin the best-conceived projections. For example, the departmental budget may allow for an 11 to 15 percent increase in supply costs. However, as the year progresses, the actual increase becomes closer to 25 percent.

Another area could be mechanical breakdowns that involve vital hospital equipment. Unexpected costs can quickly demolish a budget.

This "Miscellaneous" budgetary category serves to allocate a limited amount of funds to meet the unexpected hazards of conducting hospital business. The one obvious benefit of maintaining this category is to reduce the amount and likelihood of budgetary overruns which can be extremely unpopular with the governing board of a hospital. By doing this advance planning, those nasty surprises which can develop will not have the devastating financial impact they otherwise might have.

How do you determine the amount to be allocated to this contingency fund? As with other elements of the departmental budget, a study of the historical perspective of the department will be helpful. As an example, how much was the annual repair bill total on departmental equipment in each of the past five years? Taking an average figure and adding a reasonable inflation index factor (based on rising prices in the repair/servicing industry) should give you a fairly accurate picture of the repair costs for the upcoming budgetary year.

In addition to allowing some insurance for the surprise pitfalls, some money should be projected to meet unexpected demand for departmental services. To cite an example, expenses for a hospital pharmacy may rise dramatically if specialized medications (some of these must be flown in fresh from the manufacturer to have their maximum effectiveness) are required for patient care.

Unexpected community demands may alter the supply cost outlook dramatically. A major fire in the area could quickly result in heavy demand for respiratory therapy services for smoke inhalation cases and the supplies needed to treat burns and other related injuries could rapidly disappear.

While events of this type would result in an increase for hospital revenue figures, some temporary cash flow problems could result if some form of contingency allowance is not built into the hospital's day-to-day working budget.

In essence, the Miscellaneous Contingency Fund provides flexibility in the hospital management plan to meet the unexpected demands placed on hospital services. Meeting this challenge is the essential element in maintaining community trust and building a secure financial base for your hospital.

Developing the Total Budget

When each of your department chiefs has submitted a budget for his (or her) section, the review process by you and your controller begins. Each element of the proposed departmental budget must be scrutinized. During the review process, the controller may ask for explanations or clarifications of certain budget items from the individual department chiefs.

During a lengthy negotiating process between the controller's office and the various hospital departments, the revenue projections and the budgetary demands for hospital operations are reconciled to the mutual benefit of all parties concerned. This process ultimately results in finalized departmental and complete hospital budgets.

Due to the controller's function as the daily monitor of the hospital's financial health, the real responsibility for budgetary decisions, as much as is possible, should be left to him. In the continuing review of hospital operations, he probably has a more intimate knowledge of which budgetary levels are realistic and which are not.

After the controller has thoroughly reviewed the working operational budget for the hospital, you can productively join the process in formulating the long-range Capital Outlay Budget. Your administrative objectives and proposals, subject to board approval, will no doubt have a price tag. These figures must be compiled to give the governing board a reasonable picture of the hospital's management planning and financial stability.

Hospital Resurrection Through the Capital Outlay Budget

As mentioned earlier in this chapter, facilities can play a major role in the financial viability of a hospital. If a hospital lacks the capability to offer adequate services to a community, it will inevitably have difficulty in attracting and retaining competent physicians, surgeons, and specialists.

This lack of facilities can quickly cause the financial base of a hospital to erode, threatening the total collapse of the health care provider.

A CASE IN POINT: EFFECTIVE BUDGETARY CONSTRAINTS RESURRECT A DYING MICHIGAN HOSPITAL

One Michigan hospital faced a severe problem with the physical limitations of their facility. The problem centered around the fact that the over-30-year-old structure had not been substantially changed or modified since it was built.

This fact alone resulted in reduced capabilities because modern accreditation standards had forced certain interior changes to be made. This tended to limit the variety and quantity of services that could be rendered. Each year brought further deterioration of the hospital's financial position, making it unable to compete for and successfully recruit new doctors for a physician-starved area.

After it became apparent that the hospital faced financial collapse, the previous owners sold the hospital to a community corporation. This sale helped to set the stage for the hospital's resurrection.

Under new ownership, the hospital's Board took the first step to recovery by retaining the services of a hospital management firm. The new administration quickly discerned the nature of the problems and began taking steps to correct them.

The first step was to tighten management controls over hospital operations. A tight hospital budget, permitting only a 5 percent or less variance, was instituted to govern internal operations. This tight budget on operations permitted the administration to begin the all-important long-range planning.

With the display of solid management, the community corporation was soon able to enhance the financing options available to the hospital. As a result, plans were soon on the drawing board for a major hospital expansion involving new operating rooms, a new intensive care unit section, enabling care for more patients at one time, and a renovated emergency room.

In less than four years, this hospital, that had been near financial collapse, was turned around. Its future is now bright, thanks in large measure to the firm financial management that the new administration brought to the hospital.

The tight budget, played up extensively in the preceding case history, was the cornerstone of this hospital's resurrection. Here's why! In maintaining a tight rein on operational expenditures, the hospital was able to maintain a profitable position on the services which it offered to the community.

Internal cost monitoring processes, instituted by the controller, were correlated with the running totals of the Daily Hospital Census. If the census figures showed a reduction in patient numbers, below what had been projected in the annual hospital budget, various departmental spending cuts were instituted to reflect the smaller patient load statistics.

If the trend of the hospital census were to reverse itself later on, the budgetary cutbacks could be reinstated later in the budget year to reflect the patient load requirements. The important point to remember is that the budget must be geared to the average patient load. The failure to monitor this vital area adequately almost caused our case-example hospital to collapse.

Establishing a workable hospital budget is clearly not enough to guarantee financial success. Without an adequate monitoring of the budget, regularly conducted, the best-laid financial plans could quickly fall into ruin.

CAUTIONARY NOTE

While some question does exist about making any budgetary changes due to minor fluctuations in the ongoing hospital census, there is little question that adjustments can, and should, be made in expenditures to respond to continuing changes in hospital patient population.

This can be addressed in one of several areas within the general operational framework. One major area concerns supply ordering patterns. If the supply inventory has been maintained at a high level to meet major patient demands, reduction in purchases can help to keep inventory levels in line with projected demand. This action helps to keep expenditures down during periods of reduced hospital income. When the patient traffic begins to increase, ordering patterns can be increased to previous levels.

Employee reductions are far more difficult to implement without sacrificing essential services to the patients currently housed within the hospital. Some adjustments, prudently administered, can be done. But this shold be reserved for only major patient census changes.

Patient census patterns which appear to be persistent over a longer period would definitely require more drastic action. The major point to remember is that the patient census trends be closely monitored. If this is not done, a major financial crisis can "sneak up" on the unsuspecting hospital administrator.

The First Signs of Crisis

The old adage, "An ounce of prevention is worth a pound of cure," is nowhere more applicable than in the area of hospital management. Spotting potential sources of trouble before they can get out of hand will spare innumerable administrative gray hairs and enhance the overall financial stability of the hospital, all at the same time.

The first sign of impending trouble comes from the figures in your hospital Patient Census. If your total occupancy rate is less than what your budget might project, and if appropriate adjustments are not made, you could be in real trouble.

"Your people in charge of purchasing should be on top of the situation at all times," a successful controller stated. "If your chief of purchasing sees that things are beginning to slow down, he can't wait for tomorrow or next week to adjust his purchasing plans. He has to make the changes immediately."

The second potential sign of hospital trouble lies in the area of revenue collections. If the dollars you expect to come in don't show up, you'd better find out quickly where the source of the problem lies. The problem may be centered in the billing department. If the invoices aren't sent out, the money won't come in.

In other cases, the problem could be more complex. Bureaucratic red tape from insurance companies and government agencies could snarl the cash flow situation to an amazing degree. Short-term delays may not create a catastrophic situation. If, however, the delays are prolonged, the hospital may be required to call on its cash reserves to make necessary payments, weakening its base to cope with any emergency situations.

Whatever the source of cash flow problems, they must be monitored and a speedy resolution sought. If this is not done, serious damage can be done to the hospital's financial stability.

Third, and finally, there is the factor of staffing levels for the lower echelon positions of the hospital. Overstaffing can prove as detrimental to a hospital's financial outlook and productivity as understaffing. This may, on occasion, involve making some unpopular decisions. Nobody likes to be laid off! But, if the situation clearly dictates such a move, you must be willing to make it.

The late President Harry Truman, during his years in the White House, had a sign on his Oval Office desk which read: THE BUCK STOPS HERE. That same sign would be applicable for your desk as well.

As clearly as with any United States President, the health and vitality of the entity you govern (the hospital) depends on the administrative decisions you make. And just as clearly, you must also answer to an "electorate," your hospital's governing board. You must perform your duties satisfactorily to merit re-election.

The clearest judgment of the quality of an administrator is never made when everything is going smoothly. It is when disaster appears imminent from all corners that your leadership capabilities are truly tested. Popularity and the winning of "Nice Guy" contests must occasionally be forgotten when the toughest decisions must be made. The best measure of any decision is not its popularity, but its effectiveness in dealing with the problem it seeks to solve.

Wrapping Up the Budget Process

The final step in the budget process, the formal portion, is to get the figures organized into an understandable pattern for presentation to your governing board. Unless your figures are totally out of line, you should be able to get Board approval. If you follow the outline set out in Chapter 4, you can expect reasonably smooth sailing for your budget.

The important points to remember in presenting a budget to the board is to have complete command of your facts. Show the board comparative figures between your proposed budget and those approved during the previous year or two. If there is a marked deviation between the proposed budget and previous ones, explain why the changes were made.

If your presentation is complete and detailed, and accompanied by adequate follow-through to see that the approved budget is carried out within reasonable variation limits, you'll find that the hospital budget process will be your best management tool for internal operations, as well as a productive relationship with your governing board.

That, in essence, is the name of the game. The two-pronged approach of a formal budget *and* a close monitoring process for implementation is your best assurance that your hospital will never sail the stormy seas of administrative crisis. *

---

* More financial information may be obtained from ¶3301 *et seq.*, Prentice-Hall *Hospital Cost Management Service.*

Effective human resources management techniques

DUE TO THE LABOR-INTENSIVE NATURE of hospital services, there is probably no more important middle management position within the hospital authority structure than that of Human Resources or Personnel Director. As the crucial link between the administrator and the general staff of the hospital, the Human Resources Director (H.R.D.) serves to keep the working environment and employee attitudes in tune with the interests of maximum productivity.

Many noted industrial management consultants state that administrative difficulties increase in direct proportion to the dependence upon people to do the work. By this criterion, successful hospital administration must rank as one of the most difficult management positions you could ever find.

The intricate psychological balance between the need for certain levels of productivity and the physical and mental well-being of the employees assigned to perform the tasks is sometimes difficult to maintain. One industrial supervisor called it the "Velvet Boot Theory." "The trick," he said, "is to kick someone in the pants without letting him feel the boot."

This is the talent that is the most important prerequisite for any successful hospital personnel director. As the most noticeable authority, from the viewpoint of the employees, he (or she) is on the "hot seat." The policies and directives of the personnel director will have a direct bearing on the attitudes which employees will carry to their work. This, in turn, will have a direct effect on the quantity and quality of the work they perform.

The Personnel Director: Qualities and Qualifications

The individual in this demanding position has considerable responsibility for the attainment of your management objectives. What specific qualities and qualifications should you look for in the prospective personnel director?

Whether you promote someone from within the hospital or retain an individual from outside the present staff, the first prerequisite should be supervisory experience in some form. In having this experience, the person has already shown some ability to work with people. The level of success attained in any previous position should also be an item for consideration.

This supervisory experience also indicates that the person has leadership potential, a definite advantage for the personnel director. In addition to the recruiting function, he (or she) should also be an effective motivator of people. Enthusiasm for the hospital's management objectives should be foremost in the director's communications with new and current hospital employees.

A second job requirement for the director is to be a reasonably good judge of people and character. The quality of hospital care is hinged directly on the quality of the personnel hired to fill staff positions. Every member of the staff must be a "team player" to make optimum management objectives work. Any failure along these lines can reduce total productivity and create disruptive frictions within the hospital's staff framework.

This fact is crucial because "one squeaky wheel can slow down the entire wagon." Department supervisors, encountering an uncooperative worker, will become agitated and could begin taking out their frustrations on innocent employees. This unfortunate fact of human nature can quickly cause a degenerative effect, like a cancer, which can spread throughout the hospital.

The third, and possibly most important, job requirement is a working knowledge and skill in diplomacy. In serving as a liaison between the employees and the hospital's administration and governing board, the personnel director should assist the administrator in formulating policies which will assure smooth departmental operations and keep employee morale at a reasonably high level. This, alone, can be a major advantage in achieving your management objectives.

Formal Hospital Personnel Policies

Efficient hospital operations are largely dependent on a good relationship between the hospital's management and its employees. Maintaining consistent and fair hospital-wide policies in employee relations is a key element in keeping the work force happy and productive.

The development of good personnel policies begins with defining the rules for the 17 commonly recognized personnel policy categories. These categories would include:

    (1) Conditions for Initial Employment.
    (2) Promotions and Transfers.
    (3) Termination of Employment.
    (4) The Merit Rating System.
    (5) Employee Services.
    (6) General Labor Policies.
    (7) Health and Hospitalization.
    (8) Hospital Holidays.
    (9) Working Hours.
  (10) Sick Leave Restrictions and Benefits.
  (11) Rules for Leave of Absence.
  (12) Miscellaneous.

(13) Safety Conditions.
(14) Employee Training.
(15) Vacations.
(16) Salary and Wages.
(17) Job Analysis and Description.

Many of the items in each of the above 17 categories tend to be duplicated from one hospital to another. Due to this standardization, and in the interest of brevity, we will concentrate only on those areas for which noticeable variation might be advisable. The rest will be given only the briefest of mention, for review purposes.

(1) Conditions for Initial Employment

Due to the fact that many hospitals are unionized, the conditions for employment are usually dictated by the contractual agreement between the hospital management and its union. Union philosophy dictates that, with the possible exception of salaried professionals, layoffs and rehiring (as conditions dictate) be conducted solely on the basis of seniority. This " last hired-first fired" ethic is the rule, rather than the exception.

Occasionally, this line of thinking can run into direct conflict with the best management interests of the hospital, forcing the furlough of some extremely efficient employees. This factor also tends to diminish the authority of a hospital's administration. Due to these contractual restrictions, some extreme cases could appear as though "the tail was wagging the dog." With more militant unions, some administrators become almost afraid to act, fearing the potential of a wildcat strike.

The ideal situation, if it can be maintained, would give management the flexibility to furlough employees based, in order, on (1) qualifications for the job, (2) employee's job efficiency, and lastly (3) seniority. This order of priority would assure that the goals of maximum efficiency could be maintained.

The only sure method to maintain administrative management controls over employee activities is to reject any contractual provisions which might limit this very necessary flexibility. For the best financial and community interests of the hospital, the administration must maintain control over all aspects of daily operation.

Hiring new employees is generally considered a joint responsibility of the department chief and the personnel department. The personnel department's primary responsibility is to maintain a reservoir of suitable applicants to fill vacancies as they develop. Department chiefs are usually encouraged to actively recruit staff members, particularly if it involves individuals with professional background or skilled trade workers.

State and federal law regarding nondiscrimination in hiring practices generally regulate policies that pertain to the sex, age, religion, nationality, etc., of the applicant. Unless hiring practices would tend to develop a predominance of one particular group, no targeting of any ethnic or racial group for preference is generally advisable.

However, in a related matter, it has been found that it is poor management policy to permit relatives to work together in any department. Aside from the potential public relations problems which this appearance of nepotism might create, close relatives working together can possibly create an adverse working climate for productivity.

From the public relations angle, it is good policy to give preference to local applicants, provided that such applicants have equal or greater qualifications for the available positions.

All applicants must, of course, pass a physical examination as a condition of employment. In addition to assuring a healthy group of employees, the legal ramifications for health insurance benefits and workmen's compensation would be minimized.

(2) Promotions and Transfers

This area is usually governed by some form of in-house seniority system, regardless of whether or not the hospital is unionized. The only time this would be varied is if the individual employee's qualifications would make a variation the best course for the interests of patient care and/or hospital efficiency.

Whenever possible, higher-level jobs are given to current hospital employees, as opposed to hiring an applicant from outside. Notice of position openings are generally posted within the hospital to inform the staff.

If employees wish to be promoted within their current departments, they should discuss it with their department heads. For other departments, inquiries should be directed to the personnel department.

Any promotions that cross departmental lines become the joint responsibility of the department chiefs involved, along with the personnel director. In an intradepartmental promotion, the consultation only needs to be between the individual department chief and the personnel director.

For purposes of raises and salary standards, a new promotion is considered in the same manner as new employment, with vacation time being based on the date when the promotion was accepted. All other calculations involving the employee are based on the total seniority gained during her employment at your hospital.

In the interests of hospital efficiency, temporary or permanent transfers (if not in the nature of a promotion) may be conducted at the discretion of the department chiefs or administration. If transfers are for one week or less, pay scales for the previous position are maintained. If the transfer is for a longer period, pay scales are determined by the new position.

(3) Termination of Employment

Due to the various elements of state and federal labor laws, termination (firing) of an employee must usually have a specific, tangible cause. Discharge without cause may be a prosecutable offense, depending on the laws written in your state.

Except in flagrant cases of employee misconduct, standard procedure is to give the employee two work weeks' notice. This can be reduced to one week, if hospital conditions so dictate. Notice of any shorter duration may be compensated by one week's pay.

If employee misconduct is involved, the employee may be relieved of his (or her) position without prior notice by concurrence of the department chief and the personnel department.

Employee resignations normally carry the same time interval requirements as employer terminations. If an employee has an unexplained absence of three days or more, the staff member is considered to have resigned. Without the specific authorization of the personnel chief, no wages will be paid to a resigning employee.

Normal operating procedures preclude giving letters of recommendation (blind "To whom it may concern" documents) to departing employees. The personnel office will, however, respond to inquiries by a prospective employer.

Before departure, each employee must have a last, brief interview with the chief of the personnel office.

SPECIAL NOTATION ON EMPLOYEE POLICY

Some hospital officials question the need for solid and firm employee policies, preferring a more flexible system. While this is clearly their right, they seriously sacrifice important management objectives in the process.

Whenever a hospital employee clearly understands that negative actions will bring a definite and uniform response (in all cases), there is very little likelihood for misunderstandings. With firm guidelines, there is no room for guesswork. As a result, expectations are clearly defined and productivity naturally increases.

Without firm employee policy, you are begging for trouble. If you beg for it long enough, you will invariably find it.

---

(4) The Merit Rating System

This area of hospital-employee relations is possibly the greatest source of controversy, particularly in unionized hospitals. Under the merit rating system, a regular review of the hospital staff is conducted to determine the relative value of each employee to the hospital management plan. The evaluation, rather than the employee's seniority, is often used to determine suitability for departmental promotions, transfers, or increases in salary.

This rating is conducted by the employee's immediate supervisor. The employee is informed of this rating and his reaction to it is recorded for future reference.

Because of the relative importance of this system, any negotiations between a hospital's administration and its union should seek to safeguard this formal system of employee analysis. If this system is lost, the long-term best interests of hospital efficiency and financial stability might be sacrificed.

(5) Employee Services

Due to the standardization commonly occurring in this area, detailed discussion is not really required. This area of employment policy normally covers the subjects of employee buying privileges, lockers and rest rooms, personal mail, personal phone calls, uniforms, meals, living quarters, transportation, parking, and pension plans.

Pension plans are probably the only subject that merits any further discussion. In this area, the development of pension plans through banks and similar financial institutions seems to offer certain benefits worthy of administrative examination. An example would be the Keogh plans which incorporate high-yield bank certificates to build individual pension fund bases rather quickly. With the projected continuation of high prime rates, these double-digit builders could be a solid, insured investment for your employees' futures.

(6) General Labor Policies

General labor policies outline, in written form, solid personnel management objectives. Such objectives would include free flow of information between supervisors and employees, hospital privilege to retain the best possible personnel (either inside or outside the hospital), establishment of a grievance procedure, established policies concerning fringe benefits, and management flexibility on quantities and types of work required by employees.

In the event of policy changes, employees must be informed of their effects on the working conditions. If changes result in elimination of a position, every effort is made to retain the employee in another capacity. If termination is required, on a limited basis, the retention of any staff members will be based on their qualifications, efficiency, and seniority (in that order).

This last part, qualifications being considered first, is another point that must be retained as "sacred" from the effects of union negotiations. Administrative flexibility and the long-term financial security of your hospital depend on your freedom to retain the best suited individual for the job at hand.

(7) Health and Hospitalization

Due to the relative standarization of requirements regarding pre-employment physicals and the procedures involved during employee illnesses, no lengthy discussions on this subject are required.

State and local health codes cover most of the major areas involving employee illnesses and return to work after recovery. With only minor variables, the standard procedure for care of ambulatory employees is to provide clinical care, not requiring hospitalization, by arrangement between the administration and the medical staff. Any employee hospitalizations are the individual's responsibility.

Generally, employee health care financing is done through an available insurance or prepayment program. Participation in this type of program is usually a requirement for employment. As an added benefit, many hospitals will offer care to employees at a discount.

(8) Hospital Holidays

Hospitals, like most employers, offer six designated holidays for their employees: New Year's Day, Memorial Day, Independence Day, Labor Day, Thanksgiving Day, and Christmas Day.

Due to the variable nature of hospital employment, absence from duty during holidays may not be possible. In such cases, an alternate day off is given within two weeks of the holiday. If that is not possible, pay for holiday work is at 1½ times normal salary for the one day. This is in addition to the pay for the holiday.

Religious holidays not falling into the previous group may be observed by an employee without pay or by substituting work on one of the designated holidays. This type of holiday observance must be arranged for and approved by the department and personnel chiefs a minimum of ten days in advance.

(9) Working Hours

Standard employment procedures, 8 hours a day and 40 hours a week, usually govern hospital employment. Except in emergency cases. every effort is made to maintain this status quo. Regardless of a hospital's status regarding unions, normal meal time and coffee break procedures have proven to enhance efficiency and productivity.

These break periods are scheduled at two-hour intervals covering the entire shift. Variations may be required if emergency cases arise. No rest period schedules are permitted to interrupt the required care or the efficiency of hospital operations.

Some positions require that a staff member is "on call," even when he (or she) is not within the hospital. These "on call" periods are *not* treated as overtime work.

Overtime employment at the request of department chiefs is compensated on a time-and-a-half basis, with periods not exceeding a half-hour being given straight time status.

(10) Sick Leave Restrictions and Benefits

Sick leave benefits are built into personnel agreements as a form of financial protection for short-term illnesses which are beyond the control of the employee. Due to the potential of abuse, normal safeguards are usually instituted to insure that such benefits are not received without legitimate cause.

Within hospital confines, this safeguard takes the form of examination and authorization of the personnel health physician. No sick leave benefits are paid out without this authorization.

In cases where illness is prolonged, exceeding the allotted sick leave days, additional sick leave time is not compensated. Though this added time is usually not credited as vacation time, exception might be made if recommended by the physician, department and personnel chiefs, and approved by the administrator.

All other facets of this subject are covered by either a hospital-union agreement or the stipulations of federal and/or state labor laws.

(11) Rules for Leave of Absence

Though these rules tend to vary in different places of employment, the general objective in granting leave of absence to an employee is to assist the person in resolving any larger personal or professional problems which might adversely affect his work for the employer. Theoretically, granting a leave of absence enhances the employee's performance when he (or she) returns to work.

For example, a nursing aide might decide to further her education to join the ranks of licensed practical nursing. If she is a particularly productive employee in her current position, granting a leave of absence to permit this education might be an excellent opportunity to gain a first-rate LPN for the hospital staff.

Another example might be a major illness of a member of an employee's family. If the concerns generated by the illness adversely affect the performance of a usually solid employee, a leave of absence given for the term of the illness might serve in the mutual best interests of both employer and employee.

Requests for leave of absence must be made in writing, becoming a part of the employee's official employment record. The rules of "Acceptable Cause" for granting leaves are set by official hospital policy. The important point to remember here is that the policy is sufficiently strict to prevent abuse. Yet, by the same token, there must be enough flexibility within the system to promote the best interests of the employees and hospital management objectives.

Because this area is so variable, we will not indulge in specifics. However, any leave of absence policies your hospital currently has, or plans to adopt, must meet three essential objectives:

(1) Remove any obstacles to optimum employee performance.
(2) Assist employees' development in their current or advanced hospital positions.
(3) Permit optimum productivity within the hospital during any transition periods.

Regardless of the internal mechanics involved in granting leaves, if these three objectives are not being met by your current or projected policies, it's time to take a critical look at the mechanism. The policy might benefit from radical surgery to improve your hospital's productivity and financial outlook.

(12) Miscellaneous

This category encompasses a few of the minor standard items involved in hospital policy. Some included items would be prohibition of gratuities to employees, department-chief approval for taking any packages from the hospital building, employee smoking restrictions, the soliciting of contributions from employees, protection for employees' property on hospital grounds, and waiver of employee liability from any equipment breakage during performance of assigned tasks.

The nature of these items does not vary from one hospital to another, and therefore requires no further elaboration.

(13) Safety Conditions

Clearly, any employer is obliged to provide safe working conditions for its employees (or, at minimum, to strive to limit the inherent risks). This obligation is spelled out in numerous state and federal laws which govern all employers that have people, other than immediate relatives, on the payroll.

All injuries which cause workers to require leave from their jobs are compensated through the prevailing Workmen's Compensation Laws for your state. Three elements of internal policy are usually implemented for employees in hospitals.

(a) All accidents, regardless of severity, must be reported to the department chief involved, with a written report filed for each accident.
(b) Injured employees must report immediately to the personnel clinic provided by the hospital. Injured workers may not return to their jobs until approved by the attending physician.
(c) No deductions are to be made in seniority for time lost due to accidents.

To assist in preventing accidents and assuring the safest possible working environment, every hospital should establish an Accident Prevention Committee to monitor the ongoing safety conditions within the hospital.

(14) Employee Training

As a matter of hospital policy, continuing training and education of employees in specific job techniques and their relationship to the entire hospital operation is advisable. While this is particularly important to new employees, taking the form of a prescribed orientation program, maintaining departmental techniques through refresher courses and training in the new "State of the Art" techniques will inevitably enhance productivity and assure that current hospital standards are maintained.

These training programs are the hospital's responsibility and should be performed during working hours. If such programs are completed outside the employees' normal working hours, equivalent time off should be provided within one week of the program's completion, if possible.

All orientation and ongoing employee educational programs are the designated responsibility of the hospital's personnel department.

(15) Vacations

Policies regarding vacation time sometime vary according to employment agreements or union contracts. In terms of general policy on the subject, vacation time is often granted on the following scale:

(a) Designated department chiefs—20 working days of vacation.
(b) Assistant department chiefs and heads of major departmental subdivisions—15 to 18 working days.
(c) All other employees—2 weeks.

All other elements of the hospital vacation program are determined by internal policy dictated by the administration and the governing board. These minor variations are either dictated by their preference or by the regulations of labor laws and/or union agreements.

(16) Salary and Wages

This category provides a clear illustration of the difficult administrative balancing act which is required to effectively manage a hospital. While cost factors dictate a level of restraint in setting salary and wages, they still must be competitive with similar positions in other areas. If this is not done, the hospital has little chance of recruiting good, reliable employees.

The basic salary or wage schedule for hospital employees generally consists of five elements, which are:

(1) Salaries paid in accordance with state regulations and/or competitive considerations for similar positions elsewhere.
(2) Job evaluation plans form the basis for all salary considerations, except as modified by collective bargaining agreements.
(3) A prescribed minimum-maximum pay range is to be established for each position, depending on longevity of employee service.
(4) Schedules for any salary modifications for any classified positions should be designated.
(5) All salaries are to be determined on a total cash basis.

Provisions concerning overtime pay and other alterations are usually governed by state labor laws and/or collective bargaining agreements, requiring no further explanations here.

(17) Job Analysis and Description

As an extension of the preceding category, Job Analysis and Description gets into the specifics of the prescribed duties for each position of employment, describing the requirements for each job and the minimum performance levels expected.

In addition to assisting in the employee evaluation process, this precise definition of responsibilities serves to enhance efficiency by eliminating possible overlapping of jobs, i.e., the same job gets done twice. Wasteful duplication can quickly have a detrimental effect on a hospital's financial picture.

However, these same policies should not be so inflexible that they reduce available patient services, particularly as they pertain to their personal comfort. In some limited circumstances, a small amount of cross-training and duty flexibility could serve to enhance productivity.

As an example, a nursing aide might be permitted to replace a simple, screw-in type light bulb in a desk lamp at the nurses' station without calling the maintenance department. However, for the sake of hospital record-keeping, such replacements should be recorded with Maintenance to prevent supply inventory discrepancies.

Similar examples could be cited in numerous areas of hospital activities. A member of the housekeeping department, for example, might (if time permits) bring a new box of tissues to a patient requesting it. If a job can be accomplished without reducing the efficiency of the employee's primary job, nor have a detrimental impact on a patient's health, such minor variations should not be discouraged.

The real test of job description policies comes in their effective implementation in actual experience. If the policies serve to enhance efficiency and productivity, they should be encouraged and maintained. If not, they should be reevaluated, with changes made where effective management interests indicate.

Employee Morale: the "Bottom Line"

In implementing these various factors of administrative personnel policy in a fair, even-handed manner, the personnel department plays a major role in maintaining the productivity of a hospital's staff. The rules which serve as a framework for employee activities must be implemented equally with each worker, regardless of the employee's stature on previous jobs, possible relationships with other staff members, or other factors.

For example, an employee should not be treated any differently even if he (or she) might be a relative of a governing board member. If any employee is shown favoritism for any reason, this has a degenerative effect on the entire staff.

Open access to the personnel department is a vital point to remember in departmental operations. If your employees can conveniently and comfortably visit your personnel office to discuss their problems, the net effect will be a positive one.

Generally speaking, office layout and the forms required for recruiting new employees are relatively standardized and similar to those used by other forms of business. This is *not* the crucial element in personnel department operations.

The *vital* element in successful personnel work is to be able to deal effectively with the intangibles of human feeling and emotion, molding an effective hospital health care team that is not based solely on the paychecks that the employer delivers each week. There must also be the bond of loyalty which holds the employee to the hospital and encourages each staff member to look out for their employer's best interests.

By effectively cultivating this loyalty factor to its maximum degree, you can assure that staff turnover and its related problems will be minimized. No other factor will have a greater effect on this department's success.

A CASE IN POINT: ADMINISTRATIVE ATTITUDE CREATES CLIMATE FOR EFFECTIVE EMPLOYEE RETENTION

To illustrate this, let's consider the example set by one small midwestern hospital that has been in operation for slightly more than 20 years. During this period, it has experienced fewer than a dozen voluntary resignations from the staff (excluding those who retired due to age). Ninety percent of the current staff have been employed by the hospital for five or more years. Over 15 percent have been employed there since the hospital was opened.

What contributed to this employee loyalty and made such long tenures possible? An informal survey revealed a number of small factors that were cited by some employees. One factor, however, seemed important to almost all of the employees. They believed, through the actions of the administration and the personnel office, that the hospital cared about its employees *as people*.

One member of the nursing aide crew summed it up best when she said, "The higher-ups here don't just view us as a means to an end, only paying attention to us when there's a job to be done. We are made to feel important—not just for what we are and the jobs we do, but also for *who* we are. I wouldn't work anywhere else if the pay was doubled."

This illustration clearly shows that attitude, even more than the mechanics of the department's operation, will determine its ultimate level of success.

Unfortunately, attitude, this number one qualification, can't be "learned" by the personnel department. It must exude naturally from each individual involved. Like many hidden elements in a finely tuned machine, the operations of the personnel department are most often noticed when they are not working properly.

The Administrative Role: Some Final Thoughts

As administrator, your role becomes one of overseeing the general operation, not dealing with the daily specifics of the department. This does not, however, mean that you have no effect on their operation.

The tone of your administrative activities and *your* attitude toward department staff will have considerable impact on *their* methods. For instance, if you are always too busy to discuss problems which might arise in the department, this can become contagious. This practice may be subconsciously passed on in their dealings with the hospital staff.

If personnel department problems commonly plague your hospital, take your *first* look at the attitudes you employ in daily activities. A portion of the problem might be originating from you. *

---

* See also ¶3801 *et seq.*, Prentice-Hall *Hospital Cost Management Service.*

Profitable purchasing and materials management practices

8

WITH THE SUBJECT OF COST CONTAINMENT gaining an ever-increasing degree of prominence in today's management scenario, the duties of the purchasing department become a vital link in the management process. Because all supplies and equipment are acquired through the hospital's purchasing department, any real efforts at cost containment must begin here.

In every area of hospital operations, the work of this department is felt. If any department is running out of supplies, it is the Chief of the Purchasing Department who comes under fire. To avoid problems, this department must be properly organized and designed to operate at maximum efficiency. Often, the total efficiency of the hospital is directly proportional to the efficiency displayed in Purchasing.

In addition to the procurement function, this department must also maintain a monitoring system to be certain that adequate, but not excessive, supply inventories are maintained at all times. This balance is one of the major concerns for any hospital's purchasing director.

To serve the interests of cost containment, the ongoing supply inventory should not be greater than the use projections for the average patient load reflected in the hospital census. Excessive purchasing can tie up vital hospital resources long before they would otherwise be needed.

On the flip side of the coin, vital supplies that are not present when needed can easily create a crisis situation. Inadequate catheterization supplies, for example. could prove life-threatening in some cases. Innumerable other examples could be cited which would illustrate this same situation. There is, however, no room for dispute as to the possible detrimental effects of a vital supply shortage.

Striking an effective balance between these two opposite extremes is the primary responsibility of the Purchasing Director.

Defining Purchase Department Responsibility

Depending on the policy set up by the hospital's governing board, the authority of the purchasing director may be fairly restricted or of broad scope. Whichever might be the case for your hospital, the levels are set according to five definable criteria. They are:

(1) Purchase Centralization.
(2) Board-granted Authority.
(3) Vendor Selection.
(4) Quantity Decisions.
(5) Cost Factors.

For purposes of review, let's take a brief look at each of these five areas to refresh your memory on the fine points of the operation.

(1) Purchase Centralization

The level of purchasing centralization that each hospital utilizes is most often dictated by the governing board. The board, for example, may decide to permit some individual departments, such as dietary or x-ray, to do its own purchasing.

A serious case could be made for permitting individual department heads, particularly those with very specialized needs, to conduct their own purchasing. As an example, the dietician, due to her greater background and knowledge on food values, might well be the better choice for food buyer than the purchasing director. Yet, because of the time pressures and possible procedural shortcomings, the converse might also be true.

If we would have to state a standard rule on the subject, the best rule of thumb might be: "Maintain a centralized purchasing function unless the proposed decentralization would contribute to efficiency and/or enhance the level of patient care."

IMPORTANT POINT TO REMEMBER ON SPECIALIZED PURCHASING

While it is true that hospital purchasing departments can characteristically handle routine purchases for most departments, there are definite instances where specialized knowledge is required to make an intelligent purchasing decision.

As an example, if a sales representative were to present a new innovation in radiology technology to the hospital's purchasing manager, the purchasing manager might not have a full appreciation of the potential benefits which could result from a purchase. On the other hand, the radiologist might quickly see the value of making the purchase.

In cases such as this, we would recommend that the department chief (in our example, the radiologist) be permitted to authorize the order—provided that this falls within the department budget as approved by the administrator and the hospital board of trustees.

If the purchase would mean additional expenditure, in excess of the projected budget, the action would then be required to pass administrative and purchasing department approval. In any event, the purchasing department must be notified of the department chief's actions to maintain proper purchasing records.

---

(2) Board-granted Authority

As mentioned earlier, the authority of the purchasing director can be extremely variable. At some hospitals, provided the budget is adhered to, the purchasing section has virtually a free hand in making purchasing decisions at almost all levels. In other cases, the authority is extremely restricted, requiring board approval for almost everything but the most minor purchases.

Most hospitals operate somewhere between these two extreme positions. The governing board, in determining purchasing policy, often reaches its decision based on how much it trusts the administrator to monitor this vital function.

The *average*, and probably most prudent, purchasing policy permits purchases of routine supply items and smaller equipment to maintain efficiency, provided that the purchases are made within the confines of the current budget.

Board policy will usually dictate that larger items, with a specific dollar limitation, require board approval before purchases. This moderate governing policy has the advantage of maintaining administrative flexibility to meet hospital needs while, at the same time, permitting the board to maintain control over capital outlay expenditures that might not correspond with community interests and desires.

This form of checks and balances, while sometimes presenting the frustration of formality, must be classified as a necessary evil. Since the governing board still retains the legal and moral obligation to monitor the hospital's management, it must maintain some mechanism within policy to be certain that this legal authority is not circumvented or abridged by administrative action.

(3) Vendor Selection

Because most hospitals represent a very lucrative market for the supply companies, there is considerable competition to get your business. Who does get your hospital's business? How is this decided?

Whenever possible, most hospitals like to rely on local vendors and supply houses to acquire institutional necessities. The cost considerations can sometimes cause variations in this plan, particularly if there is a major price differential involved. Except in cases where bids are involved, requiring specific Board approval, general hospital policy is usually the guide for these considerations.

In addition to giving preference to local suppliers and a bid policy, other areas of policy may restrict the number of suppliers to cut accounting costs, give preference to firms which have proved accommodating during hospital financial troubles, using technical and advisory services that some suppliers provide, maintaining in-house testing services, and setting up quality specifications for all hospital supplies.

These policy decisions have a direct and profound effect on the operations of the purchasing department. In most cases, the guidelines and controls play a beneficial role. If, however, the policies are inordinately restrictive, the necessary flexibility for effective daily hospital management may not exist.

The usual case is to develop a generalized framework policy which serves as a guide for the purchasing function, leaving the specifics (except for the larger items already mentioned) to the discretion and judgement of the administrator and purchasing director.

(4) Quantity Decisions

The extreme fluctuations which have become the rule, rather than the exception, in the current marketplace make any attempt to set standardized policy in this area counterproductive. Changes in suppliers' marketing strategies can often result in different buying patterns to gain maximum advantage of price schedules.

As an example, purchasing 1,000 of an item, as opposed to 500, might result in a 20 percent or greater per unit cost savings. If usage projections and expiration dates for supplies don't dictate restraint, ordering the larger quantity can result in a substantial financial advantage.

Often the greatest constraining factor in larger quantity purchasing lies in the speed of obsolescence for hospital technology. "Sometimes," said one hospital official, "an item becomes obsolete a month or two after we get it."

Scientific advances, particularly in the area of medical and surgical technology, happen with such frequency as to render long-range planning virtually impossible. Supply and equipment manufacturers play a large role in this problem, discontinuing the production of necessary supplies for older equipment as newer technology comes to the marketplace.

Supply house and vendor representatives often get some advance notice as to changes in product lines, new equipment to be introduced, etc. In discussions with sales representatives who visit your hospital, the purchasing director may be able to get a reasonably accurate picture of the short-range future to assist in purchase planning.

The obsolescence factor, along with standard inventory requirements to assure efficiency, will usually be the best guide in the quantity decision-making process.

(5) Cost Factors

The final, but possibly most important, criterion in any purchasing decision is the *actual cost* of the item in question. By actual cost, we don't mean the price set by the manufacturer, supplier, or vendor.

Actual cost, in this context, is applied to the total costs incurred by the hospital in utilizing the product. In computing this actual cost, a number of hidden factors must be examined, analyzing their impact on the management picture.

For instance, if new equipment is purchased for a hospital department, how much will it cost for training and orientation to assure proper equipment use and maintenance by departmental staff? Is this factor negated by the long-term gains in efficiency? Will the department register financial gain by utilizing the newest equipment available? If so, can this gain be specifically quantified? Will the quality of performance be enhanced?

In the area of supplies, numerous other factors must be considered in determining actual cost. These factors might include accounting costs, work hours involved in receiving, record-keeping, and merchandise inspection, time involved in actually using the item, patronage refunds, transportation charges, and the esthetic values represented by product use.

In both areas, such factors as product obsolescence, manufacturer and supplier guarantees, availability and cost of outside repair services, and storage costs must be considered in the final purchasing decision.

If the final actual cost becomes prohibitively high, the best policy is to refrain from making the purchase, regardless of how attractive the supplier's offer might seem on the surface. This analysis will help to prevent serious management errors that could result in financial difficulties for your hospital.

Monitoring Quality: An Important Function

One very important factor in enhancing efficiency and the quality of hospital care is being sure that the quality of supplies being used meets hospital standards and the purchase specifications used in making the buying decision.

The purchasing department should coordinate in-house testing procedures to evaluate such areas as camouflage, chemical content, construction, thread count, color fastness, design, flexibility, performance, heat resistance, size, tensile strength, durability, eye appeal, weight, and general safety features.

If all incoming supplies are faithfully monitored, there is little chance for a dishonest supplier to pull the wool over the eyes of an unsuspecting purchasing director. This monitoring process will assure that the high standards of hospital care and general operations that the community has a right to expect will be maintained.

Basic Supply Management Regulations

The avoidance of supply shortages is a major concern for almost every business. This is particularly true in hospitals. As mentioned earlier, a shortage could quickly result in a crisis situation.

Therefore, it is vitally important for every hospital to set up a mechanism for continuing inventory monitoring and supply re-ordering to prevent shortfalls. An 11-step plan is generally recognized as being the most effective in maintaining effective supply management controls.[1]

The 11 plan elements are:

(1) An initial inventory, including quantities and values of all supplies on hand, should be set up.
(2) As new shipments arrive, all items should be recorded in the ongoing inventory process.
(3) Departmental requisitions should be used to acquire supplies from the storeroom.

---

[1] For further information, see PURCHASING AGENT'S DESK BOOK, Janson, Prentice-Hall, 1980.

(4) As requisitions arrive, needed shipments should be made to the departments involved promptly.

(5) Stock records should be maintained for all items currently on inventory. When items are delivered on requisition, the appropriate adjustments should be made on applicable cards.

(6) If items requisitioned are not in stock, the requisition form should be returned to the department placing the order, stating that the desired item is on order or has never been stocked in the storeroom. In the latter case, purchase orders should be issued for the approval of the purchasing director.

(7) When supply shipments are received, as per the purchase order sent, the storeroom clerk should review the items received, with comparison to invoice, for quantities, grade, price per unit, and the total price. If correct, the invoice should be forwarded to the business office for their action. The storeroom clerk should also submit a receiving report, signed to designate approval of payment to the supplier or vendor involved.

(8) One day each week should be specified for the receipt of the weekly stockroom requisition by the storeroom clerk.

(9) Emergency requisitions should get priority handling and delivery.

(10) All employees should be given detailed instructions as to the appropriate use of supplies. This serves to cut down on waste and prevents unintentional misuse of some supplies.

(11) All supplies, whether received or issued, should be checked carefully.

These 11 detailed steps in the storeroom management process, if faithfully implemented, will serve to assure that, from the supply perspective, high levels of interdepartmental efficiency are maintained.

As a general rule, the less complicated a system is, the easier it is to administer properly. For the sake of simplicity, the barest essentials of record-keeping require that *three* types of forms are maintained. They are:

(1) The purchase order.
(2) The store requisition.
(3) The continuous inventory system (stock record cards).

Some other forms, suggested by management consultants as being desirable, include a purchase record, purchase requisition, quotation request, delivery receipt, record of goods received, return order record, and a detailed report on overage items, shortage, and damage.

Computers: The "Short Cut" Method to Ordering

An interesting development in the purchasing area has come through the effective "marriage" of the computer and the telephone to enhance the speed of conducting most hospital transactions. The system involves the use of a punch card which is, when completed, inserted into a small terminal attached to the phone system.

The Data Card provides columns on which item numbers, quantities, and other pertinent information are recorded by punching out the appropriate spaces on the card. When this card is fed into the terminal, the card is scanned and information transferred along the phone lines to the supplier. Transactions which commonly took several minutes to conduct can be completed in mere seconds with this system. The savings, in long distance phone charges alone, can be considerable.

To get a clearer picture of this situation, let's take a look at the system in action.

A CASE IN POINT: NEW SYSTEM REVITALIZES EASTERN HOSPITAL'S PURCHASING DEPARTMENT

With an ever-increasing burden imposed by labor costs and the inherent cost of maintaining large inventories, one eastern hospital sought an innovative solution to bring these costs into line.

After detailed analysis, this hospital chose to incorporate a punch card system for ordering proccsscs. Using this system, they were able to substantially reduce the necessary revolving inventory required to maintain essential hospital services.

In addition to the reduced inventory, the purchasing department was able to reduce its expenses by an amazing $50,000 in the first year, more than paying for the system's installation and implementation costs. This ongoing system's operation is expected to yield over $500,000 in savings within 8 years.

The net effect of this type of program can be very dramatic, effectively reducing delivery time on most essential supplies (provided that suppliers are connected to this system also). While the system has not been in existence long enough to ascertain its longevity (the ability to perform without mechanical breakdown), all current indications point to favorable results.

As the utilization of computers is expanded in the business realm, this system will undoubtedly become quite widespread, enabling most hospitals to use it for the vast majority, if not all, of their supply transactions.

Computers and Inventory Control

Expanding on the idea of computer utilization a bit further, their use in the area of inventory management and control has become an increasing factor in the essential procurement decisions being made by many businesses and professionals. Hospitals, though somewhat slower about making the transition, have made considerable strides in this area during recent years.

The greatest advantage with computers lies in their capacity to maintain ongoing inventory analysis as a vital part of their daily function. With computers, supply departments can keep running totals on all items which leave the storage area. This makes the development of accurate Use Projections fairly easy. When these usage figures are used prudently, they can be an effective means of determining needed quantity purchases. This can help the purchasing department to make needed adjustments in buying patterns, long before they can have an adverse effect on the financial stability of the hospital.

This can be extended even further by programming the computer to "flag" major changes in Hospital Census figures, warning the purchasing department to make the needed alternations on time. The computer, if used properly, can become an excellent ally in effective hospital management.

Group Buying: An Effective Alternative

As the effects of inflation become an increasing factor in hospital management, new ideas to combat this potentially crippling problem have been initiated. One of the most promising alternatives in current use is the combined purchasing agreement, commonly referred to as Group Buying.

The method described in Chapter 3, combining the purchases of a hospital and its doctors, is a form of this arrangement. This idea, though effective, merely serves to illustrate the proverbial tip of the iceberg in terms of the potential for its application. When applied on a massive scale, some fairly impressive results can be expected.

To effectively implement this type of arrangement, three essential elements must be a part of the initial planning. They are:

(1) Effective purchase planning within each individual hospital.
(2) Good communication between participating facilities.
(3) A pre-established central clearinghouse-type facility to receive and dispense all supplies to participating facilities.

When a group of hospitals get together, pooling their financial resources and their supply needs, their ability to negotiate favorable purchasing agreements with suppliers is greatly enhanced. Because large quantities can be delivered to one place, cutting the amount of expense involved, suppliers will often return a sizable portion of the cost savings to the purchaser in the form of discounts, rebates, or some other form of inducement.

To illustrate some of the favorable results which can be obtained with this idea, let's take a look at two cases in which group buying was implemented.

CASE #1: BUYING GROUP REAPS SUBSTANTIAL SAVINGS

Faced with major supply cost outlays, four midwestern hospitals, all located within a 50-mile area, decided to get a group buying program started for their facilities. Tapping the resources of the largest hospital's purchasing department as the centralized clearinghouse for their program, they began negotiating for more favorable deals from their suppliers.

As a result of skillful negotiating and the effects of buying as a group, they achieved savings ranging from 15 to 25 percent, depending on the items involved.

CASE #2: MANAGEMENT CONSORTIUM SLASHES COSTS THROUGH THE GROUP BUYING IDEA

Capitalizing on the fact that more than a dozen hospitals were under the indirect control of one main office, a management consortium that operates in eight different states decided to get their costs into line by combining the purchases of all involved facilities into one buying plan.

After some initial analysis, the management got the plan started. The effects of the implementation were immediate and profound. In contrast to an ever-increasing supply cost per patient statistic, the new plan offered an *average 21 percent cut* in the cost of all supplies needed for all participating hospitals.

These figures are not so incredible or unique. The increased efficiencies for the suppliers provided by group buying, along with the business tradition of offering larger discounts for major quantity contracts, were the factors that made the group buying plan work.

Though the group buying idea is becoming increasingly popular, it is unlikely that the positive benefits will be canceled out by changes in suppliers' corporate policies. Discounts are simply good business for the suppliers. They will not risk losing your business by eliminating the benefits.

Group Buying: The Legal Obligations

The greatest impediment to successful implementation of group buying plans often lies in the necessary *legal agreements* which are needed to insure maximum effectiveness. Because the best buys are most often offered on long-term commitments, each hospital in a group buying plan (particularly applicable to a small regional group) must make a definite commitment, bound by legal documentation, to the purchasing arrangement. Whenever supplies or materials of any sort are contracted for, as a group, the participating hospital which ultimately is the recipient must be legally obligated to bear the costs.

This can become the greatest source of dissension among participating hospitals in a group buying plan. Because the contractual obligation is made by the group, rather than by the individual hospital, other hospitals in the buying arrangement could become legally liable to compensate for the default of one hospital.

Participating hospitals must have legal protection against this potential problem. We definitely recommend consultations with a competent business and commercial law attorney before proceeding with the formal formation of the group buying plan.

As a final legal thought on group buying, you should also consider the possibility that you may find the plan unsuited for your hospital's needs. You may want to get out! Will the final plan allow for smooth transitions when a hospital wishes to discontinue the arrangement? Or, will your hospital be tied into an unworkable plan—with uncooperative partners—which could have a detrimental financial impact?

The entire subject of group buying is complex, laden with potential pitfalls that could prove disruptive to the normal flow of operations. However, with proper guidance from legal advisors and shrewd business acumen from your purchasing department, this concept could open doors to effective cost control, an essential key to the effective management of your hospital.

The Purchasing Department: Some Final Thoughts

In the final analysis, any effective cost control mechanism that your hospital might wish to institute must be effectively administered *here*. There is no way that you, as administrator, can be at every point in the hospital at the same time. Your purchasing department manager must know the essential principles involved in daily operations, plus the legal considerations involved in the more complex forms of hospital transactions which his department may be called upon to handle.

While complete familiarity with all aspects of the hospital's operations is a valuable asset for the head of the purchasing department, the greatest single attribute that every successful director must have is an unwavering dedication to quality. Without this, the overall standard of care within your hospital can be adversely affected.

As administrator, your task is to inspire and seek to maintain the necessary dedication within the entire purchasing department. If you can succeed in this effort, you can be reasonably assured that the interests of your hospital will be served satisfactorily. *

---

* See also ¶8001 *et seq.*, Prentice-Hall *Hospital Cost Management Service.*

Effective medical records management: key element of hospital efficiency

IN TERMS OF THE EFFICIENCY AND QUALITY of the care delivered by any hospital, the key element to success is the swift, accurate, and efficient dissemination of information on patient statistics and the particulars regarding an individual's health status while hospitalized. As it applies to the area of so-called "crisis care medicine," swift information transfer to physicians and nurses could literally determine the fate of the patient.

This information dissemination, however, is only half the total picture for the functions of a hospital's medical records department. The other half comes in the monitoring function for the *quality* of medical and surgical care which has already been delivered.

As you may recall from our discussion of the Medical Records Committee of the medical staff in Chapter 3, Part 1, the detailed records maintained by this department serve a vital role in the internal monitoring process that helps to assure optimum health care delivery by every member of the hospital's medical staff.

Due to the extensive regulations imposed on the hospital health care delivery system, this monitoring system is not only advisable, but a mandated part of the hospital accreditation process and participation in the insurance benefit programs under Medicare and numerous other insurance carriers. These benefit programs form a vital portion of the revenue received by many, if not most, of the hospitals in the United States.

This chapter, offers a detailed breakdown of the function and objectives of the Medical Records Administrator, analyzing the position, and offering some specific management techniques to make departmental operations perform at their maximum efficiency.

Medical Records Administrator: Center of the Action

As the central dispatch point for all medical information needed within the hospital, the Medical Records Department is the cornerstone of efficient activities by the medical, surgical, and nursing staffs.

114

This central point for the written information regarding hospital activities should be headed by an individual who is trained in the intricacies of the medical records library. This library is the storage and retrieval point for the records needed in daily operations.

In addition to the medical records for each patient who enters and leaves the hospital, this department serves as the central processing point for many vital hospital records which are designed to improve the administrative monitoring of institutional activities.

Due to the convergence of these multiple responsibilities, the medical records administrator should have a solid command of three essential areas: (1) Library Science, (2) Management Objectives, and (3) Medical Terminology.

Departmental Operating Objectives

Essentially, the operations of the medical records department must be directed to meet five areas of hospital operations. These are:

(1) Patient Care.
(2) Medical and Related Education.
(3) Research.
(4) Legal Considerations.
(5) Administrative Monitoring, Planning and Control.

In each of the five above-mentioned areas, there has been a major expansion of detail required. Many of the major advances in medical science within the last three decades have come from the study of detailed records of past performance. These advances have, in turn, contributed to the proliferation of medical records and added importance to their existence within the hospital management scheme.

Though we have differentiated these five items for the purpose of study, it is the net impact of the whole operation that is the true measurement of departmental effectiveness and success. Each element, like a pigment on an artist's palette, serves to enhance the impact of the complete picture. No single element makes or breaks the operational scheme. But a missing element will weaken the effectiveness of the total impact.

(1) Patient Care

From the minute that a patient is admitted into the hospital, the function of the medical records department comes into play. The first step comes at the hospital's admitting office. Here, the patient (or a close relative) provides the necessary preliminary information that will become a part of the permanent in-hospital record for the patient while he (or she) is hospitalized.

This preliminary information would include such items as patient name, address, insurance information and personal data on the patient. This is followed by the formal assignment of a room for the patient.

Generally, this admission process is preceded by a physician's examination of the patient, either in his office or in the hospital's emergency room. The physician's signed authorization form is often considered a prerequisite for admission. The only exception is when physicians phone in their authorization on some cases.

These phoned-in authorizations must be followed up by a formal written authorization, signed by the admitting physician when he subsequently visits the hospital. For the sake of legal considerations, this format does not permit variations. Without the doctor's signature, both physician and hospital could become liable for damages and also be unable to collect any legitimate payments from the patient's insurance carrier.

After the patient has been officially admitted, the physician or a member of the hospital's staff, in most cases, a nurse, will begin the process of collecting pertinent facts on the patient's medical history. This information will be combined with the results of the physician's examination, assisting in the diagnostic process.

THE MULTI-PURPOSES OF HOSPITAL RECORDS

The detailed records of every facet of examination, diagnostic procedures ordered, and results obtained are used in the physician's justification for any treatment ordered for the patient. Internal hospital policies usually require meticulous records in this area because, as you may recall from Chapter 3, they serve a central role in care evaluation by medical staff committees.

In addition, these detailed records serve as a legal safeguard for both physician and hospital in the event that a dissatisfied patient files a lawsuit. Without these records, neither physician nor hospital would have any tangible evidence which could serve to refute the patient's claims.

As the patient's hospitalization continues, added notes are made concerning his (or her) progress under treatment. This is coupled with recording any patient education that is provided by the hospital and the results of the post-treatment evaluation. This final evaluation is the last step prior to the patient's discharge from the hospital.

For the duration of the patient's stay, there is an ongoing evaluation of the records sent in to the medical records department. They are checked for completeness, coded for retrieval purposes, indexed by categories, analyzed, combined with other reports from different hospital departments (as they apply to the individual patient), and filed together for each individual patient.

This continuing process simplifies the post-treatment evaluation conducted by the medical staff committees, making all necessary information readily accessible to those who need it. By maintaining this procedure, the efficiency and quality of the hospital's health care delivery system are greatly enhanced.

While the overview presented here may seem to be an oversimplification of the department's total operations, it does contain the essential elements as they directly pertain to the immediate needs of patient care.

(2) Medical and Related Education

As mentioned in the opening of this chapter, many of today's numerous scientific advances in medical care have been based on previous experience. For this reason, prolonged storage of medical records provides an excellent informational base for the physician.

For example, if a doctor is faced with an exceptionally difficult case, he may recall a similar set of symptoms from a patient who was successfully treated some years ago. In retaining old medical records, the hospital provides a research tool for this physician. By reviewing a case history that was similar, he can make some valid comparisons to increase his chances for successful treatment.

The maintenance of detailed records also permits the hospital's staff to make comparisons between those patients successfully treated and those who were not. This comparison will help all hospital staff members to prevent any potential errors in procedure or judgment, thereby improving the success rate for the hospital.

The educational benefits of medical records are even more apparent in hospitals affiliated with physician or nursing education. Patterns established by successful procedures which are documented by actual cases tend to carry greater credence with the student than mere dry facts from a textbook.

The detailed birth-to-death analysis of the human condition brings to life the mysteries of the anatomical sciences. Much of the material which is currently available for medical and nursing students, plus those training for allied health professions, has been based on the analysis of failures and successes as chronicled by medical records.

In the final analysis, the greatest contribution of medical records comes in the continuing education of currently practicing physicians and surgeons. Though no one can discount the element of human error, any added knowledge which past history can provide will serve to enhance the length and quality of life for the patients they serve.

(3) Research

As society at large and, more specifically, the medical profession demand answers to the complex and baffling illnesses which still plague us, the importance of research will continue to grow. A vital part of the research process is the scientific documentation presented through medical records.

From the initial research stages conducted in the laboratory, the detailed records of each step in the research process serve to prove the results obtained and disseminate this information for wider public benefit. The final proof of the research's value is its successful application to human anatomical sciences.

This final step, documented through medical records, serves as the major factor in the procedure's adoption for regular use. Scientific standards for evaluation of all available data require this detailed record-keeping.

We could cite numerous examples of this process in action. For example, open heart surgery, considered routine today, had its own period of infancy. From the initial laboratory experimentation with animals to the first successful application for the repair of human heart damage, the research and recording process helped to remove the potential for problems during the post-operative period, as well as to refine the operative techniques involved.

Cancer research is yet another area which could be cited for its progress. Though major strides in cancer therapy have occurred, making (at the time of this writing) numerous forms of cancer controllable or curable, there is still much work to be done.

There is little question as to the quality of the research being conducted in every hospital across the United States. As each case is successfully completed, new elements of the age-old mystery of human health are discovered. Every hospital, both large and small, serves to contribute to this vast pool of knowledge. The thoroughness of medical records that each hospital keeps will determine the value of its contribution to the knowledge of disease and human health.

(4) Legal Considerations

With the rising specter of malpractice litigations facing physicians and hospitals alike, the value of the medical records system is being put to the test as never before in history. Serving as the documentary backdrop to an ever-increasing number of court cases and hearings, the *written proof* of a physician's and hospital's activities is a vital element in preventing these lawsuits from being successful.

Incomplete record-keeping procedures can have a devastating impact on doctors and hospitals, forcing many malpractice insurance carriers to drastically increase their rates. If records had been complete, many malpractice claims might have been defeated. The sad truth is that *personal memory is not admissible as evidence in a court of law*.

A CASE IN POINT: THE PREVENTABLE $500,000 MISTAKE.

Consider the dilemma that faced a hospital and physician in the western U.S. A patient filed suit against both doctor and hospital in a case where surgery was performed that, by some standards, could have been considered an elective procedure. As a result of the surgery, the patient claimed, nerve damage caused partial, but permanent, paralysis of her right leg.

In a pre-trial hearing, the doctor testified that the nerve damage was present prior to surgery. However, no entry of this was made in either the doctor's patient record or that of the hospital.

With no documentation to back their case, the insurance carriers recommended that both doctor and hospital settle the case out of court. The final settlement resulted in $250,000 being assessed against each defendant in the case. That's a solid *half-million dollars* lost because inadequate medical records failed to protect the two defendants against the legal challenge!

Someone had to absorb that $500,000 loss to the insurance companies. Ultimately, these losses are passed on to the policy holders in increased premiums. Whether your hospital carries liability insurance or not, there is no question that inadequate record-keeping will cost your hospital money.

In every area of hospital management, the adequacy of your records will determine your ability to withstand legal challenge. But, in no other area is the need more critical than in medical documentation. From the area of civil litigation which we just covered to the part medical records play in assisting criminal investigations and justice proceedings, the direct connection between medical records and the legal community is continuous.

As medical technology becomes even more advanced, this alliance will become even closer. The questions raised by life-sustaining devices were highlighted by the national spotlight gained in the case of Karen Ann Quinlan. Numerous other cases could be cited where the advance of technology raised large legal questions that only complete medical records could help hospitals answer.

Unmistakably, the importance of medical records will continue to grow. The greatest challenge facing hospital medical records departments will be to cope with an ever-increasing amount of required paper work to meet the legal demands that federal and state legislation, plus bureaucratic regulation, will seek to impose on the American hospital health care industry.

(5) Administrative Functions

In the last category of medical records department objectives, we must give careful consideration to the role departmental activities play in assisting your office in administrative planning, monitoring, and the control of hospital activities. Without the needed information on what is happening within your hospital, how can you possibly plan for effective daily operations, much less the long-term picture of your facility?

Within the context of our earlier discussion on medical staff activities (in Chapter 3), substantial emphasis was placed on administrative participation in the medical staff's organizational framework. However, if this participation is not based on solid and available information, it is ineffective and basically worthless to your management objectives.

The information source which you must depend on to make important administrative decisions is the medical records department. With a hospital's primary objective being the delivery of quality medical and surgical care, your decisions must be geared to first serve this main aim.

After you make and implement an administrative decision affecting the medical aspects of hospital operation, the medical records department's information can assist you in monitoring the results. With your personal anaylsis, coupled with consultation with the medical staff, you can judge the success (or lack thereof) of the implemented programs.

If, as may occasionally be the case, a move proves to be counterproductive, the cumulative statistics that are compiled by medical records can point out potential problem areas as they begin developing. This ongoing monitoring process, along with medical staff consultations, is the main safeguard you have in your administrative arsenal to prevent major troubles from erupting.

These same records can spot major shortfalls in hospital capability which can prove costly in terms of lost potential income. As an example, if a larger number of cases must be referred to another hospital for further treatment, most often due to inadequate facilities or lack of a competent specialist to deal with a problem, these patient transfers result in a loss of hospital income.

A CASE IN POINT: RECORDS ANALYSIS OPENS DOOR TO MULTIMILLION DOLLAR REVENUE SOURCE FOR MIDWESTERN HOSPITAL.

One midwestern hospital came to recognize a substantial public need for kidney dialysis services within its area. Due to lower demand, these patients had been referred to a regional hospital that was approximately 100 miles away.

When the hospital's medical records began to indicate that patient numbers would be sufficient to support a local dialysis program, making it cost-efficient, the administration and the board of trustees initiated the program.

Though the initial investment in equipment and additional staff was rather high, the added $1.2 million in annual revenue for the hospital was a welcome addition, making the kidney dialysis service one of the most financially beneficial elements of the hospital care program within three years of its inception.

Without the vital statistics presented in its medical records, this hospital's administrator would not have been able to predict the beneficial financial impact that the dialysis program would have. Because the facts on patient numbers requiring such treatment clearly showed the need, this shrewd administrative decision was not a case of dumb luck.

The figures contained in the common hospital patient census are not sufficient basis for solid administrative decisions. You must also know what types of treatment appear to be most in demand. This information is only available through a detailed evaluation of your hospital's medical records.

"Written Records": The Efficiency Robber?

Accuracy in the transcription of medical records is an area of vital concern to many hospital records administrators. The problem centers around the often unspoken ire over illegible handwriting which some physicians turn in to the medical records department. This dilemma has even resulted in humorous cartoons being published in some medical journals.

The lost efficiency due to deciphering efforts done by medical records department personnel is, however, no laughing matter. As an example, recording uterine surgery on a male patient can be a source of considerable embarrassment and the need to "explain how it was done." Please don't laugh! A case like that did happen!

One effective solution being adopted by an increasing number of hospitals is to pack small cassette tape recorders on each doctor's medical chart rack that is used during daily ward rounds, the minimum once-a-day examination of hospitalized patients. Rather than write their findings, they dictate them onto the cassette.

Though the success rate for this system varies according to the hospital system in use (and the conscientiousness of the physicians involved), most medical records departments have compiled a 15 to 25 percent prodcutivity improvement when this innovation was adopted. Without the time required to decipher some poor penmanship, records transcribers can quickly bring the patient's records up to date.

This increased productivity also means that the hospital can have more patients in for treatment without increasing the staffing requirements in this department. Whenever you register a reduction in the cost per patient figures, you enhance the viability of the entire hospital.

Computers: A Revolution in the Making!

It's been called the "Computer Revolution." The electronic age which brought major innovations to the business world in general has come to the area of hospital management as well.

The cost factors which made computerization prohibitive for all but the largest corporations has been reduced as dramatically as the physical size of the units. While the early "electronic brains" were monstrous in their dimensions, the newest models have brought vast capabilities to units that aren't much larger than a standard typewriter.

The secret behind this revolution lies in the technological developments regarding micro-circuitry which enable the computers to perform many functions from a circuit board that is smaller than a poker chip. This advanced technology has resulted in a 90 percent or greater cost reduction for computerization (based on matching capabilities of today's models as opposed to those during the early days of computers).

Their use in medical records management is becoming greater as these computerization costs continue to decline. The best part of the "Computer Equation" comes from the reduced space that medical records require for storage. The contents of one filing cabinet can be reduced to a computerized disc that is no longer than the reel from a standard movie projector.

The speed of information retrieval is also dramatically increased. Hospitals which are wired for the new VDT's (code lettering for Video Display Terminals) can relay necessary information from the records department to the nurses' station needing it without either party leaving their posts. Procedures previously requiring ten minutes can be complete in a mere ten *seconds*.

Using the computerized system, medical information is automatically filed as it is being transcribed, in effect removing one step from the records management system, physically filing the papers into the cabinet.

Cost effectiveness is one primary consideration in any administrative decision. From all indications, the computer is very cost effective. In a national survey of hospital operations using computers, an average 8 percent cost reduction was registered for the hospital's record handling process. This figure included the monetary outlay involved in the purchase and installation of the computers.

**A CASE IN POINT: NORTH CAROLINA HOSPITAL PROVES COMPUTERIZED
RECORD SYSTEM FEASIBLE AND COST EFFECTIVE.**

One North Carolina hospital, wishing to improve its record transmission system and intra-hospital communications systems, set up a network of short-haul transmission computer terminals around the hospital, more than 70 of them in all.

Despite the initial setup costs involved, the increased efficiency from computer use made this extensive system *pay for itself in less than a year*.

While the current pricing schedules in the computer industry still make the units most cost effective for the larger hospitals, enabling them to use the units to their total capacity, a continuing decline in start-up investment and operations costs could bring computers within reach of the majority of hospitals by the end of the 1980's.

Due to the proliferation of computer companies and their associated vendors, the process of shopping for a computer can be a confusing endeavor. As a general rule, the established computer companies (those with the longest track records) will probably prove to be the best sources for equipment.

The only real shadow on the management picture for computers is the factor of the high prime lending rate. If the money needed for computerization must be borrowed, the interest rates might serve to wipe out the potential gains you might enjoy.

The scenario currently painted by most economic analysts points to a continuation of high interest rates for a prolonged period. This sour note is the one element which could remove computerized medical records management as a viable option for all but the largest hospitals considering such a move.

Medical Records Management: Some Final Thoughts

Because the medical records department serves, in effect, as a clearinghouse for your hospital's records, we have not covered the specific forms generated by each department that contribute to the medical records workload. Instead, we sought to provide the outline of a departmental management plan which works.

Aside from that, we also addressed some specific problem areas where the medical records department could get into trouble. Some of the innovative solutions which have been reported in this, and preceding, chapters have worked for other hospitals.

These potential solutions are only a starting point for your analytical processes. The real essence of problem solving for medical records management, as it is for all other areas of the hospital, is to look for the *two* levels of solution.

First, you look for the easiest method to remedy the *immediate* problem, in effect, to "stick your finger in the leaky dike." But this only serves to prevent the problem from growing to unmanageable proportions.

The second level of solution lies in looking at the *possibilities*. This is the area that yields the best long-term results. By asking what can be feasibly attempted to address the problem, the *permanent solution* for most management problems can be found. *

Perhaps the best management advice comes from the echo of a 1968 Presidential campaign speech by Robert Kennedy when he said: "Some men see things as they are and ask 'why?'. I see things as they could be and ask 'why not?'."

---

* See also ¶8301 *et seq.*, Prentice-Hall *Hospital Cost Management Service*.

Essential steps for organizing effective engineering and maintenance services

THANKS TO THE TREMENDOUS PROLIFERATION of advanced technology in hospital operations, the role of maintenance and engineering services has become a source of great concern for most hospitals today. The reliance on technology has made effective maintenance and engineering practices a vital cornerstone for most aspects of daily operations. If equipment or machinery is not working, the activities of a hospital can quickly grind to a halt.

To assure that this does not happen in *your* hospital, the maintenance activities must be based on the most current technological information available to the head of the department. A continuous process of training in new equipment standards and repair procedures is an imperative to keep most repair activities an internal hospital function, a vital element in keeping standard upkeep expenses for advanced technology to an absolute minimum. As we will review a bit later in this chapter, reliance on outside repair personnel can prove to be prohibitively expensive for most hospitals to consider.

The road to achieving this objective must be based on solid organization for maintenance services and the allied engineering functions of the hospital. We will discuss this, along with ideas for keeping proper control mechanisms working efficiently and in the best interests of the department and the hospital.

And finally, we will discuss some potential solutions to the greatest sources of concern in maintenance and engineering management. The solutions offered could have a dramatic effect on the overall cost picture for your hospital.

Departmental Organization and Staffing

The chief operational cog in this department has customarily been referred to as the Plant Operations Supervisor, the title serving to encompass the large variety of activities involved in the job. If anything goes wrong with any piece of hospital equipment or any portion of the hospital facility, the plant operations supervisor is the individual who hears about it.

124

In larger hospitals, this function is divided between two people to assure 24-hour-a-day coverage of all equipment with the best trained hands available for emergency repairs. The absolute minimum standard for any size hospital is two maintenance persons. This permits on-site coverage on both day and afternoon shifts, with the night shift being covered by a rotating on-call status.

Though few experts pinpoint an exact staffing level for a hospital's maintenance department, the level of work encountered at most hospitals would indicate a minimum requirement of one staffer per one hundred beds of hospital capacity, with a minimum of two (as indicated earlier). Depending on the level of technology used in the hospital and the number of external maintenance agreements being utilized, this staffing requirement number might be forced higher. In some cases, as we'll discuss later in this chapter, a larger maintenance department could result in markedly lower costs for all general maintenance and repairs and could be, as well, a major promoter of hospital efficiency.

The major element of importance, regardless of the numbers involved, is to have adequate training for all maintenance staffers—with special emphasis on the training and qualifications of the plant operations supervisor. For this reason, the trend in recent years has been to retain a graduate engineer for this crucial hospital position. Though this would represent a short-term increase from the hospital salary viewpoint, the staffer's increased training would result in a decreased reliance on outside maintenance services, a major cost cutter if implemented correctly.

For the plant operations supervisor, the interconnecting lines of communication would be to the administrator, the business office, and with almost every department chief within the hospital. By passing along any pertinent information about equipment acquisitions or other aspects of facility management, as instituted by the departments involved, the plant operations supervisor can be certain to have his equipment and maintenance files accurate and current to aid his work.

Considering the supervisor's background, a sound administrative argument could be made for consulting him *before* any major equipment purchases are made. There may be pertinent engineering considerations which would make some purchases definitively counterproductive from a cost and overall efficiency viewpoint.

Recorded Information Promotes Efficiency

As an effective basis for maintenance operations, the hospital's plant operations supervisor should always maintain a file of maintenance schedules, electronic schematic diagrams, and mechanical manuals or guides for every piece of equipment owned by the hospital. From these informational tidbits, a solid program of preventive and rehabilitative maintenance can be developed.

In addition, his office should house the working drawings and floor plans for the hospital, showing structural specifications, foundation plans, wiring and plumbing information, ventilation system specifications, and the layout for storm and sanitary sewer lines.

With all of this information on file, the plant operations supervisor has a satisfactory base to enable him to prevent major problems of a mechanical or structural origin as well as to limit disruptive effects from the problems which do occur. This is essentially the main objective for the maintenance department.

The hospital's reliance on utilities, mechanization, and electronic equipment is so complete as to effectively disrupt any rational efforts at clinical or administrative activity. In short, if a serious breakdown in a hospital's technological system occurs, orderly operations can quickly disintegrate into chaos.

This reliance also precludes a system of temporary repairs, most often found when maintenance departments are inadequately staffed in quality or quantity to get the jobs done. While the "quick fix" can help to push ahead the ultimate reckoning for a short period, it also can set the stage for major problems in the future. What happens if all of the "temporary" repairs break down at the same time?

Rather than being caught in a situation of being "Penny wise and Dollar foolish," the objective of the maintenance service should be to invest small amounts in preventive work on equipment and facilities instead of being forced into major outlays for large-scale repairs.

By emphasizing the preventive program, a hospital can realize major savings in the capital outlay sector of its budget by reducing the need for larger amounts of back-up equipment to cover potential breakdown periods. An efficiently operated maintenance department could reduce equipment expenditures by 20 percent or more by two different avenues; (1) extending the life of all equipment currently in the hospital's service, and (2) reducing the need for replacement parts through effective preventive maintenance procedures.

Internal Department vs. Contract Services

During the past 15 years, there has been a dramatic increase in the number and variety of companies which offer maintenance services (at a price) for a hospital. While this trend proved to be significant in the reductions of administrative concern, contract services have ultimately been perceived as a two-edged sword which can hurt, as well as help, a hospital's operations and financial outlook.

After the inflationary pressures began having a major impact on our society in the mid-1970's, the hurting edge of the contract services question began to manifest itself. As in anything purchased from an outside firm, the service provider's profit is its primary concern. When the cost factors for providing services increase, this is automatically passed on to the purchaser. For the time a hospital retains an independent firm to provide maintenance services, the costs are not under the direct control and influence of the Administrator.

Except in the cases of purchasing "Extended Warranty" for equipment items as part of a general manufacturer's purchasing agreement, the servicing firm has no great financial incentive to be conscientious about preventive maintenance services. Unless contrary provisions are written into the service contract, the providing firm might be financially ahead by letting your equipment or facilities fall into slight disrepair. A major fix-up job could be charged to your hospital, above the normal fee charged for standard maintenance services.

Though this idea might seem unethical, particularly to the victimized hospital, these service providers are counting on the "Time Factor" to work in their favor. When a portion of your facility or a piece of equipment suffers a breakdown, you want the problem taken care of RIGHT NOW. Admittedly, you're in a very poor bargaining position during a time of crisis.

Because you don't have time to get another servicing firm to do the job—without creating cirtical gaps in patient care services—you merely shrug your shoulders and attempt to make the best of a bad situation. When everything is running smoothly again, the tendency is to gloss over the difficulties which you encountered and proceed without making any major changes.

This is precisely the attitude which the service provider (with marginal ethics) expects from you. It is the number one reason that *he can stay in business.* If you, and other administrators retaining his business, refuse to accept this situation and demand changes, the marginal operator faces two choices. He must either clean up his act or go out of business.

By contrast, an internal hospital maintenance service comes under direct administrative control. The service's employees are retained specifically to be certain that no major breakdowns occur. Their job continuity depends on being successful in this goal.

The time to press for constructive and financially beneficial changes is during periods of smooth operation. If your hospital is currently dependent on outside maintenance sources for a major portion of its needs, we strongly urge you to begin making the transition to an in-house service now. Though you can continue to maintain a connection with factory repair people for some equipment (it's financially beneficial during warranty periods), all other repair and maintenance duties should gradually be transferred to an in-house program.

Major Savings Through In-house Maintenance

Though most hospitals do not rely exclusively on outside maintenance firms for services, the common rule is a hybrid combination of a limited in-house service and specialized maintenance services from a commercial outlet. While this arrangement might prove beneficial for equipment with potentially hazardous components (x-ray and radioisotope equipment are examples), limiting a hospital's liability toward its in-house staff, the basic maintenance schedules for all other equipment in the facility should be handled by an in-house staff.

Repair costs, when such events occur, can be kept to an acceptable level if handled by a competent staff of hospital maintenance people. The combination of a reduced tangible bill plus the major reductions in equipment down time which result from having an in-house repair technician available can offer substantial savings in the hospital equipment budget.

To underscore this point, let's take a look at one maintenance program which achieved good results.

CASE IN POINT: WESTERN HOSPITAL SAVES 35 PERCENT ON ANNUAL MAINTENANCE AND SERVICE BILL

As the costs of contracted maintenance and repair services continued to escalate, one western hospital decided to make the transition to an in-house maintenance and repair program to replace the excessively expensive contracted services agreement which had been in place.

Though the service agreement had worked fairly well for this 200-bed facility, the $30,000+ price tag annually was more than the administration was willing to accept. Beginning a gradual transition to an in-house program, retaining one full-time repair technician and a part-time technician, the services were transferred to the in-house program as each individual service contract expired.

While some noticeable results were apparant immediately, the first full year of operation under the complete in-house maintenance and repair service was most revealing. During the first full year, the costs declined from the previously mentioned $30,000+ cost to just under $20,000 per year, a cut of over 35 percent.

The other major benefit of the program was a dramatic reduction in equipment duplication to compensate for down time, the cut totaling over 20 percent. The first year savings from this source alone was almost $100,000. These savings converted a projected budget deficit into a small surplus.

The action taken by this western hospital clearly illustrates the importance of getting a handle on the major problem of maintenance costs. Rather than being faced with a potential rate increase, which would be frowned upon by hospital regulators, this hospital was able to regain control of its own destiny through solid and decisive action.

Likewise, your hospital could dramatically turn its fortune around using this same principle. By not overlooking a hidden source of excessive spending, like this one, severe budgetary imbalances which have often served to increase hospital rates can be avoided.

Hospital Maintenance and the Energy Question

Like every other business in America, hospitals have felt the severe squeeze of the country's energy situation. As large-scale energy users, hospitals have suffered from the increases in rates for everything from electricity to natural gas that have escalated their operating costs by dramatic amounts. Cost containment objectives dictate that the vigilant hospital maintenance service take a direct role in fighting back against the energy price menace.

Though the structural integrity of a hospital does play a major role in energy use, the maintenance service should also become involved in the direct monitoring of energy use by all staff members and equipment. Besides analyzing the energy requirements of all equipment which is purchased by the hospital, their efficient usage should also be taken into account in any effective energy utilization planning.

A new trend designed to help maintenance departments to handle this large job is to utilize a network of microcomputers to handle the monitoring function. The computer system has proven to be an excellent investment for the hospitals which have instituted the program. As a descriptive example, let's take a look at one medium-size hospital which installed computers for the monitoring function.

CASE IN POINT: WESTERN HOSPITAL PARLAYS $30,000 INVESTMENT INTO MAJOR ANNUAL ENERGY SAVINGS PROGRAM

In direct response to a rising energy bill, one western hospital decided to put its maintenance service in charge of monitoring the facility's energy use. Because of the extensive nature of the monitoring function for this medium-size hospital, a microcomputer system costing almost $30,000 was installed to assist in the process.

Using a system of automated on-off interconnection, many pieces of hospital equipment were automatically turned off when they were not in use. Though there were manual override provisions for the equipment to be used when needed, the result of this monitoring process by computer quickly became evident.

Thanks to the computer system's watchfulness, the hospital's energy bill was slashed by 30 percent per year. This represented a total payback for the system in two years or less.

This case study clearly illustrates that a hospital, given proper equipment and the determination to take the appropriate steps, can fight against supposedly fixed expenses which can irrevocably lead to long-term financial problems, and possibly even the collapse of the entire health care delivery system.

With the continuing escalation of energy costs, which seems inevitable under current economic and political conditions, along with the current of international events in major oil-producing regions, your maintenance service could play a major role in the continued financial health of your hospital. *

Departmental Control Mechanisms

Aside from the incoming records mentioned early in this chapter, the maintenance service is also subject to a small amount of outgoing paper work. The main objective of these written records is to assist in administrative monitoring of departmental functions. This would include periodic reports to the administrator, parts and supply requisitions, inventory listings, and detailed cost analytical material.

While this material is sufficient for a maintenance service that is appropriately operated, these records would not reflect the hidden costs of equipment problems, including lost time by hospital staff members and other residual inefficiencies which breakdowns inevitably create. Also unlisted are hidden costs to patients who may require increased hospitalization because the quality of care might have suffered.

---

* See also ¶6501 *et seq.,* Prentice-Hall *Hospital Cost Management Service.*

From the administrative viewpoint, the shortcomings of these flat statistics should definitely be recognized. Some analysts have estimated that the combined effect of tangible and hidden costs in equipment down time can represent over 20 percent of a hospital's total budget. Though we might consider this to be a *slight* overstatement of the case, we definitely agree that these hidden costs should be considered in any analysis of the maintenance service.

Closing Thoughts on Maintenance Services

Throughout this chapter, the prevailing message has been the necessity of an efficient maintenance service to the future viability of a hospital. Few experts on hospital management would consider disputing this fact. Setting administrative priorities to gain this objective can be somewhat trickly considering the unpredictable nature of the service's function. There is little likelihood that equipment malfunctions can be predicted with complete accuracy. The same statement would apply to structural aspects of the hospital.

The main objective of a hospital's maintenance program should be to minimize the risk. By keeping a reasonably tight rein on standard equipment surveillance, minor problems can be picked up and corrected before they can evolve into the catastrophic efficiency-robbers.

If your maintenance service keeps things moving appropriately, their records will reflect a very high proportion of their activities being devoted to minor repairs, insufficient to cause disruptions in vital patient services. This proportional analysis between minor and major repairs may be the best way to judge the effectiveness of your hospital's service.

Provided that this balance can be positively maintained, with very few noticeable disruptions, you can be reasonably assured that your hospital's maintenance service is working to further the best possible operations of your facility. *

---

* See also ¶6201 *et seq.,* Prentice-Hall *Hospital Cost Management Service.*

The hidden links to hospital efficiency

11

BENEATH THE VISIBLE SURFACE of daily hospital activities, there are operational areas which generally remain unnoticed *unless they are not working*. These important links to hospital efficiency often are overlooked by the public and, all too often, by the hospital's administration.

Three hospital departments generally meet this rather ignominious fate; (1) the Housekeeping Department, (2) Laundry and Linen, and (3) Hospital Security. Yet, without adequate and efficient operations in any of these three areas, the effectiveness of the hospital's service to the community could be adversely affected.

In this three-part chapter, we will delve into the operational standards and requirements to make each of these three areas efficient and coordinated with the other functions of the hospital.

Part 1 will examine the organization and operations of the Housekeeping Department. As part of this review, we will look at staffing requirements, responsibilities, supplies, and training. In addition, a discussion of the department's responsibilities during fire and evacuation procedures will be included.

Part 2 will involve information pertaining to the efficient operation of the Laundry and Linen Department. The discussion will include organizational fundamentals, facility requirements, and a method to accurately predict the staffing needs for the department.

Also included will be a discussion of methods to improve productivity through personnel techniques and innovative auxiliary marketing for laundry services. These can prove very beneficial in maintaining cost containment goals for laundry and linen operations.

From the viewpoint of economic advantage, we will also have a detailed review of the in-hospital laundry vs. shared laundry services, pinpointing specific new innovations that might prove additionally beneficial if the laundry service is modified.

131

For those hospitals which prefer contract service laundry to an in-house setup, we will offer specific guidelines to avoid problems in hospital supply, with an analysis of when conversion to in-house facilities might be warranted.

Part 3 covers the fundamentals of hospital security service planning. Fundamental security policy, procedures, and the service's central role in fire safety and evacuation planning will also be discussed.

The section will also feature detailed ideas on police procedures which should be incorporated into hospital security services, particularly in the larger metropolitan areas. This would especially apply during periods when prisoners or other potentially violent individuals require hospital care.

And finally, we will offer some ideas on sharing hospital facilities with local police agencies in an effort to improve hospital security and virtually eliminate the need for specially trained security personnel on the hospital's payroll.

PART 1—HOW TO DEVELOP AN EFFICIENT HOUSEKEEPING DEPARTMENT

Housekeeping duties in a hospital, as in almost every home, go basically unnoticed unless they are left undone. A clean house is essentially taken for granted. The same applies to a clean hospital. Cleanliness is the expected normal condition.

The hospital's housekeeping department, centrally responsible for maintaining this normal condition, operates in the shadows of other hospital departments. Functioning in a peripheral fashion, avoiding clashes with essential patient health care functions, the department's duties center on general cleaning and hospital germ control. The most visible point of the department's function comes in room preparation between the time when one patient is discharged and another is admitted.

Infection control procedures throughout the hospital are a direct responsibility of the housekeeping staff, which uses cleaners and disinfectants to maintain sanitary conditions. This emphasis is particularly important during the warm summer months when a large variety of bacteria, most notably staphylococcus, are present in numbers that present a danger to patient's health.

The winter months also represent a challenge in the form of various viral infections. Limiting the spread of influenza and pneumococcal viruses definitely requires extensive and thorough sanitation procedures. Even under the best of conditions, these infections can present a serious challenge to a hospital's capabilities to handle them effectively.

Having the appropriate organizational and procedural mechanisms in place, along with solid training concepts for all housekeeping staff members, will help assure that the functions of the department will be performed in a suitable manner.

Housekeeping Staff Structure

As with other distinct hospital departments, the housekeeping service has a designated head whose role is supervisory to the staff as well as being responsible to the administrator for the proper performance of designated duties. Unlike other hospital departments, it is unlikely that there would be an authority substructure for the housekeeping service (with the possible exception being the extremely large facility).

The Head Housekeeper (chief of the department) should have a fairly solid background in the areas of home economics and physical sciences, particularly as they apply to the department's activities. Detailed knowledge of active properties of cleaning agents and other supplies being used is a prerequisite for their intelligent purchase and use.

Because the usual housekeeping staff is basically an unskilled group, the head housekeeper should also be competent in conducting an ongoing training program for the staff to promote the best possible operational practices and limit departmental waste.

Staff Training Programs

Unlike the majority of a hospital's departments which require skilled personnel at almost every position, the housekeeping service contains the largest proportion of unskilled labor. This fact necessitates, as mentioned earlier, an ongoing program of training for staff members.

Depending on the skills and expertise of the head housekeeper, this training can range from on-the-job supervision to a detailed classroom-type training program. The classroom program, in combination with supervision to limit the development of bad working habits, has been judged to be the most effective means to accomplish desired goals.

The classroom program can be developed effectively through the use of available audio-visual materials, used in combination with direct instruction by the head housekeeper. Many training programs also utilize a measure of written material which is handed out to housekeeping staff members for their study.

The greatest benefit of formal training programs appears to be the enhanced feeling of professionalism which is generated. This greater confidence translates into motivated action on the job.

Staff professionalism also creates another positive byproduct: major reductions in staff turnover. This is a natural part of the process. If an individual feels greater satisfaction at the job she is doing, it is unlikely that she will want to leave.

Detailed training also helps to eliminate major sources of waste created by uninformed product usage. Because the emphasis during daily operations is on getting the work done, there usually isn't time for the employee to stop everything and read the container's label for usage instructions.

The training program's purpose in this area is to instill this necessary information into the employee's memory, making the process of following appropriate instructions automatic rather than a matter of conscious thought.

To illustrate this, let's look at a case study of housekeeping staff performance after a detailed training program was instituted.

CASE IN POINT: EASTERN HOSPITAL SLASHES WASTE THROUGH HOUSEKEEPING STAFF TRAINING PROGRAM.

With its increasing staff turnover rate and supply waste becoming ever-larger factors in housekeeping operations, one eastern hospital decided to try a detailed training program for the housekeeping staff.

After sending the head housekeeper to a training seminar to enhance her skills at teaching her employees, the hospital established a strong program of audio-visual and coordinated written material to assist in the staff training program.

Almost immediately, the noticeable effect of the program was professionalism. Rather than "dragging around" at their jobs, housekeeping staff members approached their work with a higher level of enthusiasm. Because the importance of their function was emphasized in the program, the employees began to feel more like integral parts of the management objective. This change in psychological conditioning also made staff members more receptive to the information regarding procedures which were offered in the training program.

The results of the program speak for themselves. As the program progressed, staff turnover was reduced by a remarkable 69 percent. Other results included:

- Cleaner usage—down 24 percent.
- Floor stripper use—down over 50 percent.
- Floor finish use—down almost 50 percent.

Though the supply use was cut so dramatically in these and other areas of the service, no reduction in performance quality was registered. This reduction was merely an *elimination of waste*.

Considering the fact that such a large percentage of supply use was purely a matter of waste, the cost of the hospital's initial investment in training materials and equipment was quickly returned in the savings generated by enhanced efficiencies. The training program could definitely be considered a positive investment for any hospital having problems with housekeeping.

The Team Concept

During the process of staff training, the head housekeeper also has the opportunity to instill a feeling of "Team Unity" in the employees. While the daily processes of cleaning are generally a matter of individual effort, these can be translated—at least on a psychological basis—into a matter of team performance.

By developing the idea of a housekeeping team, the total performance of the staff will become a matter of *individual* pride. This individual pride translates into a form of internal monitoring system for the staff, helping members to motivate each other to better performance. This idea could also be bolstered by incentives to employees for slashing waste or better productivity.

These incentives could further bolster the team idea by being based on the total performance of the staff, not on one individual's contribution. This would set the stage for a bit of friendly competition to see who could contribute the most to the team's goals and total management objectives.

As you can see, this idea, particularly as it applies to the housekeeping service, is a psychological trick to gain maximum performance on a prolonged basis. While this would not represent any major investment, only a form of "sharing the savings," the effect could be a major contribution to the overall cost containment objectives you wish to maintain.

Housekeeping's Fire and Safety Duties

As the caretaker for a hospital's cleanliness, the housekeeping department also has a peripheral, though equally important, role in maintaining safety standards for the hospital. This would involve the development of procedures for all flammable substances in the domain of the department.

With an increasing reliance on potentially flammable chemicals in cleaning agents, appropriate storage procedures are an absolute requirement for insured safety. The same idea applies to paints used in the hospital. Paints and oils are not allowed to be stored in any buildings housing patients.

Any form of aerosol spray container must be handled with considerable care, and stored in relatively cool areas. The potentially explosive propellants used in these containers can present a distinct hazard if not properly stored.

As a final item, any potential hazards spotted by housekeeping staff members, but not under their direct jurisdiction, should be reported to the department responsible for its rectification.

In the event of fire, the housekeeping department's role in evacuation procedures should be firmly delineated by hospital policy, preventing any overlapping which could cause inefficiencies during a critical time. Most commonly, housekeeping personnel would assist in escorting ambulatory patients, particularly those who are not connected to intravenous devices, to safety.

Housekeeping staff might also be included for the evacuation of bed patients, serving in an assist function with nursing aids and regular nursing staff. This part would require some coordinated planning with the head of the nursing staff to prevent duplications that could prove detrimental.

While some planners might advocate limited duties in fire containment for the housekeeping department, a possibility with minor fires, the primary objective should be patient evacuation and preventing panic to assure everyone's safety.

Though fire containment functions might help to limit potential property damage until firefighters arrive on the scene, the dangers imposed by inadequate staffing for evacuation procedures would tend to outweigh this short-term advantage.

Housekeeping Functions: Some Closing Thoughts

At the beginning of this department's section, we tended to assert the hidden nature of the department's activities. The real test of housekeeping's success in a hospital's management scheme comes from how smoothly it correlates its activities to those of other hospital departments. Basically, if there is no visible reason to notice your housekeeping department's functions, you can be reasonably assured that the job is getting done.

In some hospitals, the greatest departmental correlation for housekeeping comes with the Laundry and Linen section (the subject of our next chapter part). With the maintenance of a Central Linen Room, the control of hospital linen is often delegated to the housekeeper.

For this authority alignment, the head housekeeper must also maintain connections with the business office, to get information on the daily Patient Census. This helps to prevent inefficiencies and waste in the distribution of linens in the hospital.

In some cases, a hospital sewing room is maintained to handle linen repairs and to judge quality for any continued service. If linens are judged to be unsuited to continue their primary function, they might be recycled into cleaning rags for the housekeeping department. This in-house recycling can represent a substantial savings as opposed to purchasing rags especially for the purpose. (Rags can cost 50 cents to a dollar per pound, possibly more in some areas.) Considering the amount of rags which most hospital housekeeping services use up, this can represent a substantial factor in the departmental budget.

CASE IN POINT: RECYCLING PROGRAM SAVES HUNDREDS OF DOLLARS FOR MIDWEST HOSPITAL.

In one midwestern metropolitan hospital, the housekeeping service was faced with a major shortage of cleaning rags for their work. Unable to buy adequate supplies, even at rather inflated prices, the head housekeeper began exploring other alternatives. She discovered a "gold mine" right at the hospital: worn-out hospital bed sheets.

Developing a correlated program with the approval of the laundry manager, the head housekeeper initiated an inspection program for linens as a part of her department's regular duties. When a sheet showed sufficient wear to be unsuited for its primary use, it was set aside from the regular laundry load.

After approval of the laundry manager, the sheets were cleaned separately and sent to the "Recreational Workshop" maintained by the hospital for its long-term patients. There, the sheets were cut up into appropriate size for rag use.

Thanks to this innovative program, the recycling yielded over $800 in the first year of operation. When the program was fully integrated into the hospital's operational system, this figure increased by more than 50 percent, with the savings exceeding $1,200 annually. This was in addition to providing some worthwhile activity for the patients' workshop and enhancing the ongoing program for monitoring hospital linen quality.

In terms of the multimillion dollar budgets which are common for hospitals today, the savings represented by this idea may not seem to be of major significance. But the principle which the case study illustrates is very important.

Though the savings of over a thousand dollars may be only a drop in the bucket, even in terms of the housekeeping department's budget, saving a percentage point or two in a variety of areas throughout your hospital can amount to a major sum in your total budget.

Using innovative ideas and feedback from this department, your hospital may discover methods to slash operational costs by major amounts. Open lines of communication can yield major benefits for your hospital.

PART 2— MANAGEMENT GUIDE TO LAUNDRY AND LINEN

Few hospital departments or services are the subject of more criticism from patients and staff alike than the Laundry and Linen service. As the apparent first priority for patients' comfort, the presence of clean sheets (or the lack thereof) is an item by which most patients tend to judge the competency of the hospital.

Likewise, the appearance of employee's uniforms, often the direct responsibility of the hospital's laundry service, reflects on the quality of care which patients expect to receive during their hospitalization. Staff members wearing crisp, clean uniforms inspire confidence in those around them as well as in themselves.

Though these factors may not seem as tangible as the main clinical aspects of hospital care, the positive psychological impact of personal comfort for patients is as important to the healing process as any other in the hospital's full range of services.

The full implementation of effective management for this area involves a combination of sufficient supplies, adequate staffing, and effective distribution systems to assure that required linens and uniforms are at the places where they are needed.

Organization and Staffing Requirements

The methodology of organizing a hospital's laundry is generally based on the types of services offered by the institution. The laundry, by virtue of its designated activity, is a mirror of the entire hospital operation. As each new service is added to the picture, demands on the laundry increase.

The key element to organizing a successful hospital laundry lies in the selection of a trained, competent laundry manager. Using a combination of technical training and experience, a laundry manager can readily adapt his (or her) facilities and operations to new demands and maintain efficiency.

For this reason, we would recommend that your first priority here should be adequate background for the manager. If your current manager does not have enough training, sending him to a technical school for additional education would be a good investment.

Because advances in equipment and technique are being made continuously, paying for the laundry manager's membership in a laundry trade association and subscriptions to trade journals would also be a good investment. The information available from these sources would assure you that your hospital is benefiting from all available technique and technology that is practical to implement.

Subordinate staffing for the laundry is keyed to the number of services which generate work for the facility. The generally accepted minimum standard has been one employee for each 25 beds of capacity. As the number and complexity of offered services increases, the employee: bed ratio must shrink considerably.

Previous productivity studies indicate that laundry employees can be expected to handle about 200 to 225 pounds of laundry in an eight-hour shift. Even with current advances, this figure could not be expected to increase much above the 250 pounds-per-day mark.

The average daily laundry load generated by each patient ranges from 15 to 18 pounds. By taking the average figure for daily occupancy from the Patient Census, a fairly accurate picture of the workload from this source can be obtained.

Add to this the projected load generated by any surgical and obstetrics activity, an average of 25 to 30 pounds per operation or delivery. This would include soiled sheets and bloodied surgical gowns, masks, and uniforms.

Effective laundry planning should take these variables into account to avoid inefficiencies caused by shortages in linen supply. These shortages could also present adverse effects on patient care.

To take a quick overview of the planning process, let's set up a sample laundry plan, "plugging in" some statistics on which to base our conclusions.

LAUNDRY ORGANIZATION PLAN

Projected Workload Sources and Amounts

Average Daily Patient Count —	102	
Average Daily Surgical Cases —	5	
Average Daily Deliveries —	4	
Daily General Patient Linens (in lbs.)		1,530
Daily Surgical Laundry Load		125
Daily Delivery Room Laundry Load		100
Total		1,755

Projected Employee Requirements

Full Time	7
Part Time	1

In the above organization plan, we have a situation which indicates that seven full-time employees might not be sufficient to meet some of the peak demand periods for linen service. Yet, the projected work load is not sufficient to warrant an eighth full-time employee. In such cases, the part-time employee might be scheduled to work on days when there is an abnormally large laundry load.

For example, if a hospital's surgical staff tends to have a favorite day for performing operations each week, the laundry manager can channel the part-time employee's efforts to that particular day. This would also apply to any other statistically indicated peak demand periods in the laundry's operations.

Generally, the cost of laundry operations is determined by a total of four factors; (1) initial investment in equipment and space requirements, (2) required staff levels, (3) operational efficiency created by location, transportation, and expansion possibilities, and (4) the cost of supplies and maintenance.

These four factors may be affected considerably by instituting a centralized laundry operation for more than one hospital (a subject discussed later in this section). While some hospitals might, thanks to these factors, choose to send their laundry to a commercial outfit, this move may also produce problems along with its benefits.

Contract Laundry Services

Due to the capital outlay commonly required to set up a hospital laundry, some hospitals opt to send their linens to a commercial laundry. While this move would, at least temporarily, eliminate the need for capital expenditure (the only real advantage), the daily costs involved would tend to be considerably higher than those incurred through an in-hospital laundry.

The largest difference comes from the need to have more circulating linen—approximately 20 percent more—to avoid shortages which might result from delivery delays or other factors. Using commercial laundries also eliminates the possibility for effective administrative monitoring of laundry quality or control of the ultimate costs.

There is also the distinct possibility of increased linen damage through commercial laundries. This factor, coupled with the costs involved in a required "check in and out" system, might tend to eliminate any potential advantages gained by not having laundry workers on the hospital's payroll.

Basically, only the smallest hospitals (under 50 beds) might find the commercial laundry to be a viable option for their operations. The small hospital may not be able to generate sufficient capital to permit the establishment of a laundry and, in many cases, might not have sufficient workload to utilize a full-time staff of any appreciable size.

Consolidated Laundry Services

One excellent method of streamlining hospital laundry operations, particularly applicable to a group of hospitals in a small goegraphic area, is to bring all laundry to one centralized laundry service operated jointly by the participating hospitals.

The main value of this arrangement comes in major capital outlay savings which come from sharing equipment and facility space investments. Shared facilities also help by eliminating the need for part-time laundry help due to more balanced workload requirements.

Computerization also becomes a viable possibility in the multi-hospital laundry, permitting better monitoring of linen supplies. The computerized information can prove to be a major management aid for the laundry manager and the hospitals' administrators. As the following case history will illustrate, the savings can prove to be quite significant.

CASE IN POINT: EASTERN HOSPITAL SLASHES LINEN EXPENSES OVER $40,000 THROUGH COMPUTERIZED JOINT LAUNDRY FACILITY.

With a continuing escalation of linen costs as a prime management problem for one eastern hospital, the administration decided to take part in a joint hospital laundry program operated in conjunction with several other hospitals in its area. As part of the laundry program, a computerized monitoring program was instituted to monitor the linen in the system.

When the computer began feeding out information, the administrator discovered that 80 percent of the annual linen loss was due to causes other than the common wear of daily use. Armed with this information, the hospital began a detailed internal monitoring program for linen supplies. This program worked to eliminate this loss, *saving more than $40,000 annually in replacement costs*.

In addition to this service, the computerized system also increased efficiency by coordinating daily delivery amounts, basing them on daily use figures entered into the computer. This maneuver also eliminated the daily linen inventory which was routinely conducted prior to the implementation of the computerized system.

This case study represents a set of relatively simple ideas in action. But the results were substantial, removing a major administrative headache which had afflicted this hospital for many years. These monetary savings were in addition to those achieved through the move toward consolidation.

Locating the In-hospital Laundry

The common practice in current hospital design is to locate the laundry in direct conjunction with other elements of the hospital's physical plant. This helps to reduce disturbances to patients created by the common noises of laundry operation. Location adjacent to an outside wall is mandatory to permit proper ventilation of the laundry facility.

The ideal location would be for the laundry to be in a separate service wing of a hospital. But this is probably not financially feasible, particularly for hospitals smaller than 100 beds. In any event, laundry traffic should be routed to cause the absolute minimum of disturbance to both administrative and patient care areas.

Internal Features of the Laundry

Due to the nature of laundry practices, one of the prime prerequisites is that all internal surfaces be of moisture-resistant materials. If naturally moisture- resistant materials are not available, all wall and ceiling materials should be moisture-proofed.

Floors are usually made of smooth-finish concrete (or its equivalent), with a built-in sloping to permit easy drainage. This drainage is particularly important as a safety condition (preventing falls) as well as to limit potentially unhealthy conditions due to excessive humidity generated by pooled floor water.

Slatted wood platforms around laundry machines also contribute to safety, in addition to limiting the fatigue commonly associated with standing on concrete. These platforms also have a hygienic advantage of being easily cleaned and dried.

The laundry should also have a liberal supply of window area. Windows should be easily maintainable and capable of opening to 50 percent of their areas for enhanced laundry facility ventilation. This ventilation factor is particularly important to maintain healthy working conditions for employees as well as to enhance their productivity.

Good lighting, though last on our list, is probably the most important single factor in effective laundry operations. Improper or inadequate laundry lighting practices have a definitely detrimental effect on both the quality and quantity of laundry productivity. This, coupled with the proven safety value of adequate lighting, should serve as an effective argument against being overly stingy with this vital equipment resource.

For a more detailed analysis of required internal laundry features, we recommend a booklet published by the American Hospital Association titled, "Hospital Laundry, Manual of Operations."

Improving Laundry Output

Probably the most vexing problem faced by most hospital laundry managers is getting adequate production from employees to keep down operational costs. This problem is particularly troublesome in a laundry that may be marginally too large for the workload generated by the hospital. Slack times do not motivate employees to greater productivity and represent a financial loss to the hospital.

This problem has been effectively combated by administrative communications with other hospitals in the same geographical area. Through a modified service consolidation agreement, offering to take another hospital's excess laundry, two hospitals can solve their problems at the same time.

For one hospital, it eliminates the need to expand its laundry operations to maintain the efficiency of their linen supply system. For the other, it eliminates the unproductive slack time in the laundry and is a source of additional revenue to help defray the costs of laundry operation.

**CASE IN POINT: MODIFIED SERVICE AGREEMENT
SAVES TWO MIDWESTERN HOSPITALS
FROM MAJOR LAUNDRY PROBLEMS.**

When one midwestern hospital discovered a considerable amount of wasted time and declining efficiency in its laundry, the administrator began to look for productive solutions to the problem. Thanks to the ongoing communications which the administrator had maintained with other hospitals in his area, he knew about the laundry overflow problem experienced by a nearby hospital.

After a short negotiation with the other hospital, an agreement was reached to transfer the excess laundry load from one hospital to the other. This move eliminated the need for a laundry expansion which was slated to cost over $250,000.

For the recipient hospital, the additional laundry represented approximately $15,000 in new hospital revenue, virtually covering the salary of the laundry manager and the miscellaneous administrative costs involved in hospital laundry operations.

Because of the cooperation displayed by these two midwestern hospitals, some major administrative problems were solved for both. The benefits of coordinated laundry operations between two hospitals have definite merit and are worthwhile considerations for any facility that faces major problems in this area.

Final Thoughts on Laundry Operation

Throughout this section, we have attempted to emphasize ideas designed to cut the costs of laundry operations. The laundry and linen service can, if not properly monitored, add substantially to the hospital's general operating budget. The linen replacement costs cited in our earlier case study are merely one example of how the system can flounder, almost with the apparent blessing of administrative policy.

The real danger here is to continue permitting the laundry's operation to be hidden from administrative scrutiny. An administrative attitude which amounts to, "It's only the laundry," casting the department to the fringes of administrative planning, can, in the final analysis, bear very bitter fruit on the hospital's management tree.

With the presence of a skilled laundry manager and adequate administrative scrutiny of operations, the potential problems which your laundry may encounter can be analyzed and corrected before they create a major challenge to your organizational skills and the clinical mission of your facility.

PART 3 — ORGANIZING AN EFFECTIVE HOSPITAL SECURITY SERVICE

With an increasing challenge coming from our society's criminal element, general safety of the population can no longer be taken for granted. Because many administrators have recognized that hospitals are not immune from this threat, the establishment of smoothly functioning security departments has become a priority item. While this concern is presently centered in metropolitan hospitals, rising crime statistics in non-urban areas have caused a drastic reassessment of hospital security policies on a nationwide basis in recent years.

This reassessment has triggered a major interest in hospital security techniques to combat crime within hospital facilities and to insure the safety of patients during hospitalization. This security planning has taken two distinct forms, both having merits which depend on the location and financial resources of the hospital involved.

The first alternative has been to hire security personnel for the hospital, with their becoming a part of the paid staff of the facility. This alternative has been most widely accepted in larger urban hospitals because they have had the financial resources to pay the price. Security personnel on the hospital's payroll represent a substantial cash outlay and cannot be considered a feasible alternative for smaller (under 250 beds) hospitals.

The second alternative is to closely coordinate hospital security activities with local police agencies. In a somewhat radical departure from the standard hospital image, local police agencies have been invited to share facilities with the hospital, having their offices in the same building.

This method provides an excellent source of trained security personnel at little or no cost to the hospital. Assuming that amicable and constructive relationships can be maintained between the hospital's administration and the local police agencies involved, this can have a solidly beneficial impact on the financial outlook of both the hospital and the police agencies.

The presence of police or security personnel also has benefits in disaster planning, fire evacuation, and other facets of emergency procedure. Their training and experience help to cut response time when such reductions are the most critical.

Hospital-Sponsored Security

In larger metropolitan hospitals, the presence of a security staff has become a matter of the utmost importance. With a continuously staffed security department, the potential for crime is markedly reduced, along with a greater likelihood of apprehension for felons who attempt to commit crimes against hospital property. This would even include the monitoring of staff activities for illegalities which could literally bleed the hospital dry financially.

To illustrate the importance of hospital security, let's take a look at the experience of one hospital which fell victim to the so-called "inside job."

CASE IN POINT: HOSPITAL SMASHES ILLEGAL DRUG ACTIVITY WITH ALERT SECURITY DEPARTMENT.

When one eastern hospital discovered the continual disappearances of controlled substances from its premises, preliminary evidence pointed to the distinct possibility that one or more staff members might have stolen, or aided in the theft of, the substances involved.

Pursuing this lead, the hospital's security department decided to solicit the help and cooperation of staff members they could trust to conduct an undercover evidence-gathering operation to end this $1,000 per day illegal drug operation within the hospital's walls.

After two weeks, enough evidence was gathered to arrest over a dozen hospital staff members, ten of whom faced major criminal charges from their roles in the operation. After the arrests were completed, the drug disappearances stopped completely, saving the hospital almost $400,000 annually.

In a situation similar to the one illustrated above, the expenditure of $60,000 to $100,000 annually for security staff salaries could easily be justified. The halting of large-scale criminal activity quickly repays the monetary outlays involved. Because of the large amounts of drugs involved in extensive hospital complexes, the presence of security people served (in the illustrated case) a very useful function.

Organizing the Security Department

As in other hospital departments, one department staff member should be selected as the Chief of Security. The chief's qualifications, in order to best serve the hospital, should include a minimum of five years of police experience, graduation from a recognized police training school, and special training or experience in the area of drug enforcement practices.

Minimum standards indicate that security staffing should be at a rate of one security officer per 250 beds of hospital capacity. The ideal ratio would be one officer to 150 beds, if hospital resources permit. But the absolute minimum, if you wish to have a reasonably effective security service, is the earlier 250-bed figure. A larger bed capacity ratio would spread the officer's available time too thin to give adequate protection for the hospital.

Whenever possible, the security department's office should be located at the center of the hospital, giving relatively equal response time to any portion of the facility's outer perimeters. In some cases, this could present some difficulties from a clinical care viewpoint. If that is a problem, security department location should be as close to the hospital's center as efficiency objectives will allow.

Security staff members should, in addition to the usual equipment, be equipped with a pocket pager to alert them of any problems when they are away from the central office. A detailed security plan might include designated hospital zones, with the number of "beeps" issued being an immediate indication as to the location where help is needed.

Because some hospitals assign extensive fire evacuation responsibilities to the security department, locating a central fire panel in the department's office appears to be a good idea.

The central fire panel is a slightly more sophisticated advance in fire alarm systems, interconnecting all hospital fire alarm systems to one central indicator panel. When an alarm is sounded, the panel lights up to indicate the area from which the distress call was issued. The system has extensive life-saving value, as the next case study will readily illustrate.

**CASE IN POINT: CENTRAL FIRE PANEL
INSTALLATION HELPS TO SAVE OVER
90 LIVES IN HOSPITAL BLAZE.**

When one midwestern hospital renovated its fire alarm system a few years ago, the inclusion of a central fire panel in the security department's office was considered, at best, to be a novel idea worth trying.

Slightly over a year later, the installation proved its value in a dramatic way when a flash fire moved quickly to an entire wing of the hospital. When the alarm was sounded, the security staff immediately knew the area affected and headed directly to it.

With the rapid spread of the fire immediately apparent, the security staff, in cooperation with other hospital staff members, quickly evacuated the more than 90 patients who were in the most imminent danger. The last patient was evacuated from the wing *less than ten minutes before the roof collapsed*.

Fire officials said later that any delay in locating the fire and initiating evacuation procedures would have had tragic results. The central fire panel had saved over 90 lives in a few short minutes.

Though much of the destruction attributed to this fire might have been prevented if an adequate sprinkler system had been in place (not a requirement at the time of the fire), the alarm system did help to reduce the danger to the hospital's occupants.

Fire Safety Planning

In hospitals with a viable, active security department, the common sense procedure is to include the security supervisor in administrative planning sessions on Fire Safety and Evacuation planning. Because the supervisor will probably be acquainted with the newest developments in police and firefighting procedures (most often through professional associations and journals, along with possible seminars for security professionals), he should be in an excellent position to advise on the best methods to quickly and efficiently evacuate the hospital in a fire emergency.

Periodic meetings between the security supervisor and the head of the maintenance department might also be advisable, especially when any major changes in equipment or facility are being instituted. By keeping the security supervisor informed of changes which might affect evacuation methods or present new types of hazards, effective planning for emergency procedures can be maintained.

Fire evacuation planning should be developed on a somewhat standardized format, with an emphasis on stipulating primary exit areas to be used. Primary exit areas must be established to cover fires in each designated security zone of the hospital. For example, if a fire strikes in the center of the hospital, each wing should have a designated exit point which is away from the fire area, minimizing danger of smoke inhalation to patients.

Evacuation priority should be given to patients who require oxygen use, reducing the danger of explosion and patient mortality. Because pure oxygen is such a volatile substance, particular care should be taken in removing such patients from danger.

This particular point should definitely be included as one point in a comprehensive hospital Fire Safety and Evacuation Policy and Procedures Guide. For other vital policy points, you might find it advisable to discuss specifics and regulations with your State Fire Marshall. Because fire safety regulations tend to vary significantly from one state to another, the fire marshall may be the best source of information regarding elements of the law and safety procedures.

Though some businesses and public institutions often tend to view the state fire marshall's office as a nemesis, frequently maintaining an adversary relationship, it can prove to be an excellent ally in assisting the overall fire safety planning process. The real secret is to approach the marshall's office with a spirit of cooperation, not confrontation.

By taking an administrative initiative in these contacts, you also gain the "benefit of the doubt" if an adverse circumstance should befall your hospital. When an active initiative has been taken by a hospital, there is less likelihood of punitive action on fire code violations because independent—not bureaucratically forced—interest has been shown in their correction.

A meeting between your security supervisor and a representative of the fire marshall's office would help to bridge any information gaps that may have developed. From a realistic point of view, your hospital and the state fire marshall have one shared objective—the complete safety of all patients housed in your facility.

The Convict Crisis: A Matter of Violence

With an increasing incidence of prison violence, along with a corresponding escalation in other forms of violent societal behavior, hospitals are faced with the tough challenge of maintaining adequate safeguards when called upon to treat accused felons and convicted criminals. The most difficult portion of the problem is to maintain the safety and security of other patients in the hospital. If inadequate planning is currently your hospital's case, particularly if it is located near a prison facility, there is a real danger of injuries to staff and patients alike.

A hospital security department's role in this area is to develop contacts with local police departments, State Police officials, and with prison administrative staff. Through this contact, effective planning can be developed for such vital areas as guard coverage for rooms housing convicts, relationships and lines of authority between ouside police officers and hospital staff members, and special facility requirements which might be instituted to assist the prisoner security process.

One excellent method of helping to reduce these security problems is the presence of police officers on the premises as a regular part of the hospital operations. This innovation has, in many cases, eliminated the need for maintaining a separate hospital security force.

Sharing Hospital Facilities with Police

Developing an effective relationship with local police agencies, based on cooperation, can be enhanced considerably through offered space for police activities within a hospital's facilities. While there are some admitted problems which could be encountered, a very good working relationship between administration and police officials is definitely possible.

The main stumbling block to this type of arrangement lies in the attitudes which are displayed between police officers and hospital staff members. If there is a spirit of condescension displayed by the police, it can create major problems for hospital personnel. Hospital staff members who feel uncomfortable with such close police proximity may be adversely affected in their work.

If, however, a spirit of equality can be maintained between the two areas, this arrangement can offer some substantial benefits for both the hospital and the local police agency or agencies involved.

As government budget constraints grow continuingly tighter, police agencies are having an increasingly difficult time acquiring adequate facilities to maintain sufficient services in the face of increasing police service needs. By developing a cooperative agreement with a hospital regarding facility space use, the costs are cut dramatically for police department capital outlay. This one single factor has been largely responsible for an increasing eagerness to embrace this system.

With police department offices in the same building, a hospital also picks up some substantial benefits. The police presence has a very positive impact on hospital security, often virtually eliminating crime against the hospital facility.

CASE IN POINT: WESTERN HOSPITAL CUTS THEFTS OVER 90 PERCENT THANKS TO POLICE PRESENCE.

As the number of thefts mounted at one western metropolitan hospital, with its internal security manpower unable to cope with the problem, the administration sought to find new solutions to this managerial crisis.

When the local news media began publicizing severe space shortages in the police department's headquarters the hospital's administrator came forward with an offer to share an under-utilized area with police in exchange for assistance in maintaining hospital security. This proved to be an excellent bartering arrangement.

As a result of this arrangement, the hospital was able to eliminate its own security department and save the $150,000+ annually which was budgeted for the service. In addition, the presence of police manpower in the hospital resulted in a dramatic cut in numbers of thefts.

Prior to the arrival of the police department as a tenant in the hospital, an average one theft per day was being recorded. After the police assumed occupancy in the building, this number was cut to ONE THEFT PER YEAR.

The results of this program dramatically illustrate the beneficial aspects of shared facilities. These major benefits also extend to the element of handling felons and convicts, mentioned a short while ago. To highlight this benefit, let's take a look at another case study which summarizes this vital connection.

CASE IN POINT: WESTERN PRISON RIOT SPILLS OVER TO HOSPITAL CORRIDORS.

When a western state's prison exploded into a riot situation, injuring dozens of inmates and several prison guards, the situation presented a unique challenge for the hospital nearest to the prison. Facing a need to treat the injured, it was forced to deal with an extremely volatile situation which would have strained even the best internal hospital security department.

Thanks to the fact that the hospital had a shared facility agreement with a local police department, it was ready to deal with the problem effectively. As the injured prisoners were being brought in, the heated emotions which spawned the prison riot threatened to spill over into hospital violence as well.

Because the police department was headquartered at the hospital, quick response to the developing emergency was possible, effectively quelling the hospital violence before it could endanger the health and safety of hospital staff members and other patients.

The presence of police in a hospital can be a very valuable asset, particularly during emergency situations. The shared facility agreement offers the benefit of giving hospital officials access to far more security help than might otherwise be afforded by the budget. This factor alone should be sufficient to convince a financially pressed hospital, with substantial security department needs, to pursue this particular method in solving the problem.

The Staff-Police Relationship

The relationship between hospital staff and the police housed at the hospital should, as alluded to earlier, be one of relative equality in terms of general attitude. If hospital staff members hold the police contingent in awe and are unwilling to enforce hospital rules, even if the transgressor is a police officer, serious disruptions in hospital operations can result.

Ideally, the relationship should be reasonably friendly and one in which all parties feel comfortable with one another. A form of "Open Door" policy by the police can be extremely beneficial to form a constructive bond between the police tenants and the hospital.

One western hospital reported that their staff was so comfortable with the police department that hospital employees would often go down to the police station and watch the television there as they ate their lunches.

One New Mexico hospital staffer said, "We started out not being at ease with the police station here in the same building. But, as time went on, we found they were ordinary folks—just like us. Now, I don't know how we'd ever get along without them."

This is the essential key to making a comfortable transition to the in-hospital police station program. If each sector can view the other as ordinary people there to do their jobs, neither one superior to the other, the end result will be a comfortable relationship which will ultimately pay large dividends.

Video Cameras and the Security System

In some sectors, there is a "school of thought" that the new technology of video cameras offers major benefits for hospital security. While this may be of some benefit to an efficient hospital security service with an excellent response time, there appear to be more drawbacks to the idea than real benefits.

While this system permits the security department to maintain a very low profile within the hospital, this same status has a definite negative effect. Without the appearance of security personnel, the criminal element will believe that the hospital is "fair game" for any scheme they might choose to implement. They will consider the use of cameras as a signal that the security service is understaffed and incapable of apprehending them.

On this basis, we can't recommend their use as a substitute for trained security personnel, but only as an aid to established security patterns for your hospital.

Hospital Security Services: Some Closing Thoughts

While the existence of a hospital security service is not a mandatory feature of hospital management, there are solid indications that this will change in the years ahead. As crime statistics continue to escalate, many more hospitals will begin considering some form of internal security staff to keep patients and staff members safe.

Depending on the financial resources of the hospital, either alternative (private security officers or local police agency) will work reasonably well. But the internal security service has never been intended to be a replacement for local and state police authorities in law enforcement. For major crimes committed within a hospital, the best resource available is either the local police or the state police contingent. Through cooperation with these agencies, the internal security department can be an effective deterrent to crime. If you and your security supervisor can effectively communicate with local law enforcement agencies as to your hospital's security needs, the combined efforts of these two entities can be very effective.

In come cases, county sheriff's departments have found it beneficial to "cross-deputize" hospital security personnel (if their training has been adequate to qualify under state law enforcement standards). This would permit hospital security people to formally arrest a person on hospital grounds and offers legal protection against assault directed at security staff members. (This would then carry the same charge, "Assault on a Police Officer," as would apply to any other police officer.)

If the cooperation is thorough enough with all surrounding police departments, the end result will be a hospital that is virtually immune from the threat of major crime within its walls. That, in the final analysis, is the main reason for establishing a hospital security service. Your hospital deserves the best. If done properly, a security program is one way to assure this end result for your hospital. *

---

* See also ¶6101 *et seq.,* Prentice-Hall *Hospital Cost Management Service.*

Team concepts and procedures for the nursing staff

PROPER ORGANIZATION AND IMPLEMENTATION of nursing staff planning is, by most administrative calculations, a top priority item in developing the full potential of a hospital's fundamental clinical mission. To underscore this point, one physician stated: "We see the average patients, those with no developing complications, approximately five minutes a day. The full implementation of our directives, covering the other 23 hours and 55 minutes, comes from the nursing staff of the hospital. Our success as physicians is often hinged on the acumen and skills of the nursing staff that's on duty."

To organize a nursing service along maximum efficiency lines, three essential elements should be considered in the development process. These three areas are:

(1) Provision of effective centralized facilities to permit top-grade monitoring of all patients in the hospital.
(2) Providing adequate nursing staff levels to meet the demands of clinical activities normally encountered.
(3) Making adjustments to provide for specialized nursing requirements which might be needed.

Through the development of an effective liaison between the nursing director, the administrator, and the physicians' chief of staff, the maximum benefits of effective clinical administration and business administration can be welded together. Because neither of these fundamental interests is of greater importance than the other, an inherent ability to balance these interests between clinical, public educational, and economic considerations is a prerequisite to being effective in her position.

The Nursing Director

As a mainstay of the total clinical operation, every hospital's choice for this position should be a nurse of extensive experience who also has a proven ability to

150

communicate ideas and follow through on their implementation. Serving as the planner of the nursing services, her abilities will largely determine the total effectiveness of the staff.

Along with this duty, she must also serve as a consultant to the administrator on those areas which have a direct effect on the nursing service. Also included in this subject are interdepartmental activities which have an effect on the daily operations of the nursing staff. Being the head of the nursing staff, she will often get the credit when everything works according to plan. Conversely, she also gets the "heat" if the nursing services are not performing adequately to meet the hospital's clinical needs.

To condense the overall scope of the nursing director's position, the list below summarizes the essential responsibilities she will encounter.

RESPONSIBILITIES OF NURSING DIRECTOR

(1) Ongoing evaluation of nursing care for the hospital's patients.
(2) Developing and monitoring the nursing service's policies, organization, and procedures.
(3) Maintaining adequate staffing to meet needs.
(4) Establishing and maintaining effective working relationships with the medical staff and other hospital departments.
(5) Hiring, orientation, and assignment of all nursing staff members. This is to include any in-hospital internship programs for nursing personnel.
(6) Oversight responsibilities for maintaining nursing records for clinical and administrative purposes.
(7) Monitoring nursing supplies and equipment, their use, preparation, and distribution.
(8) Developing and monitoring of the nursing service budget.

While one individual can probably perform all of these functions adequately in smaller hospitals, it is common practice to appoint an assistant nursing director at larger hospitals. The assistant director will usually assume a portion of the above stated responsibilities, and will cover for the director when she is away from the hospital.

The nursing supervisors who handle the afternoon and night shifts normally have delegated responsibilities similar to the director's, making necessary decisions which might arise during their shifts. These supervisors may also be required to cover some of the administrator's responsibilities, representing him in such cases as might be necessary.

Unit Authority Substructure

Directly beneath the nursing director, lower-level supervisory personnel are appointed to handle various *units* of clinical care and/or administrative function directly applicable to the nursing staff's activities. Some examples of individual patient-care units might include the operating and recovery rooms, labor, delivery, and nursery suites, plus the pediatrics section (if the hospital makes such a separate designation).

Each patient-care unit has a designated *head nurse* who is responsible for the functions of the unit. The head nurse is responsible to the nursing supervisor for the particular shift on which she works.

Particularly true for larger hospitals, each major clinical care division has its own nursing supervisor. The designated unit head nurse is under the general supervision of the division supervisor who, in turn, is responsible to the nursing director.

Individual nurses are assigned to the unit which requires their services or, when training prerequisites would so indicate, to the areas of their individual expertise. In most hospitals, the Licensed Practical Nurse is the individual who is assigned to one of a number of available units in the hospital.

Head nurses for patient-care units are almost invariably fully certified Registered Nurses. While this might be varied somewhat, particularly if the hospital is experiencing a shortage of Registered Nurses, it is commonly considered to be inferior policy to put a Licensed Practical Nurse into such a major position of authority.

In the final analysis, the line of authority (and those who fill each designated position) are less important than the end result of the organization, the quality and efficiency evidenced within the nursing service's daily operations.

Central Location of Facilities

With efficiency as the essential watch word of nursing staff performance, an essential element of administrative policy should be to provide centralized location for nursing stations, leaving a minimum number of steps for each nurse to reach the locations where she might be needed.

To illustrate this idea, please refer to Illustration 12-1 as we continue this discussion. This is a schematic of a nursing station layout actually being used by one Michigan hospital.

In this particular layout, designed for a small hospital, the nurses' station is centrally located at the intersection of corridors leading to most of the major services provided by the hospital. Directly adjacent to the nurses' station, the Intensive Care Unit is within prompt access range of one or more nurses at all times (without making special provisions for a separate I.C.U. nurse). The section labeled A marks the location for the heart monitors.

At the rear of the nurses' station, the portion with the letter B, all patient record charts for those rooms covered by the station are located in a rack. A writing area here, as well as on the semicircular counter which serves as the front perimeter of the station, permits efficient and prompt handling of the patients' records (as requirements dictate).

On the front counter, the section labeled C, the patient-call monitor switchboard is located. Here, the ward clerk or another person designated for this purpose receives patient requests through a voice-actuated intercom system. When the patient's needs are ascertained, a nurse or an aide (depending on the nature of the problem) is dispatched to the patient's room.

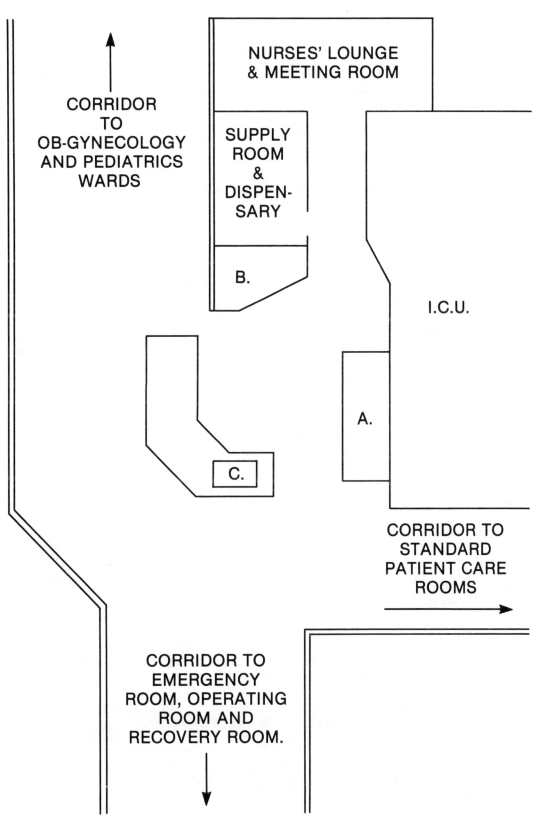

CORRIDOR
TO
OB-GYNECOLOGY
AND PEDIATRICS
WARDS

NURSES' LOUNGE
& MEETING ROOM

SUPPLY
ROOM
&
DISPEN-
SARY

B.

I.C.U.

A.

C.

CORRIDOR TO
STANDARD
PATIENT CARE
ROOMS

CORRIDOR TO
EMERGENCY
ROOM, OPERATING
ROOM AND
RECOVERY ROOM.

Illustration 12-1

More significantly, this particular nurses' station is located to provide a direct line of sight to the hospital's Emergency Entrance. Though the hospital is notified, in advance, of any ambulance arrivals, the actual time of arrival can easily be witnessed by the nursing staff at the station. By the time a patient can be unloaded from an ambulance, a nurse from this station can be at the emergency room to offer help. This line-of-sight feature is particularly important in cases where patients are brought in by car, without the benefit of advance ambulance or police notification.

The illustrated nurses' station, one of only two that serves this one-story hospital, also covers the wing that houses the obstetrics and gynecology services and the pediatrics rooms.

Though the level of activity conducted from this one station may seem to be rather extensive, the consolidation of services from one location offers the hospital enhanced efficiency by preventing an overlap of services when not required. As an example, if the general patient section is quiet, some nurses who might ordinarily be there could be called to help in an emergency in the pediatrics section. Conversely, if the reverse were to happen, a nurse from pediatrics could be pressed into service for the general patient section.

The centralized facility location permits major administrative flexibility for the nursing staff, allowing for changes in procedure without major sacrifices in efficiency. This flexibility has a positive effect on the quality of care which patients can expect at this hospital.

Within the constraints of common health care standards, this type of flexibility can also enhance the morale of the nursing staff, permitting some limited variety in the types of patients and in working conditions which are encountered. The morale factor can play a major role in the retention of experienced nurses.

Maintaining the Supply Connection

Continuing our reference to Illustration 12-1, the location of the supply room and dispensary is an important contributor to the overall efficiency of this particular hospital's nursing service. In using a decentralized system for dispensing medications to the hospital's patients, storing needed medications which do not require refrigeration, it eliminates the need for nursing staff members to walk to the pharmacy or drug room to fill each dosage as it becomes due.

The same room also houses a considerable number of other nursing supplies, cutting down the number of trips to the central supply section of the hospital. This setup serves to create major improvements in efficiency.

CASE IN POINT: NURSING STATION SETUP REGISTERS
MAJOR TIME SAVINGS FOR HOSPITAL

According to members of this Michigan hospital's nursing staff, the major problem with the average station layout is a lack of readily accessible materials, records, etc. that may be required to effectively complete designated clinical activities.

By conservative estimates from nurses who have served in other types of setups, the amount of daily walking is reduced by a minimum 30 percent, with the overall efficiency of the nursing service being improved by 15 to 20 percent.

Final Notes on the Nursing Station

While the nurses' station layout highlighted in this chapter is not the only efficient possible way to operate a nursing cubicle, the design does point out some essential basics to be considered. The real emphasis, regardless of the design chosen, should be on limiting the amount of time inefficiently used in moving from one place to another.

Also, the centralized location for a nurses' station is the second important consideration. By attempting to maintain fairly equal distances to each of the areas (the outer perimeters) which are assigned to be served by each station, enhanced patient care will be an inevitable byproduct.

When these two considerations are incorporated into your nursing service planning, you can be assured that the floor plan will be making a major contribution to the total efficiency of your hospital.

Staffing Levels for Efficient Operations

Due to the increasing demands on most hospitals' nursing services, along with a growing trend toward nurse specialization, the growth of staff requirements has been at a steady pace since the early 1960's. With growth from a range of .7 to 1.1 nurses per patient bed capacity to a range of .9 to 1.5 nurses in a period of 15 years, the challenge of maintaining adequate nursing staff levels has increased dramatically.

The problems of a shortage in new nursing graduates, combined with a high job turnover rate within the profession, has forced many hospitals to scramble in an effort to maintain adequate nursing staff levels. The complexity of today's nursing picture has resulted in an overall minimum standard of one nurse per patient bed capacity. If staffing levels were to drop markedly below this level, a definite nurse shortage could be considered to exist.

Innovative Nurse Retention Programs

With the ongoing nurse shortage becoming increasingly acute, administrators are beginning to examine new ideas to encourage nurses to locate and remain at their hospitals. In addition to heavy recruiting efforts at nursing schools around the country, some hospitals are making active efforts to entice former nurses back to the clinical environment of the hospital.

These efforts have spawned a number of solid ideas for expanding nursing staff participation in the policy-making structure of the hospital as well as new methods to reduce staff turnover rates. For the purposes of this chapter's discussion, we will concentrate on the two techniques which have displayed the greatest degree of success; (1) staff-initiated nursing programming, and (2) the nurse internship program.

(1) Staff-initiated Nursing Programs

One major problem of the nursing program in many hospitals is the removal of *personal initiative* from the professional nursing process. With the exceptions of the nursing director and, if one is needed at your hospital, the assistant nursing director, the remaining members of your nursing staff probably are not involved in the active policy-making decisions which affect the daily operations of their department.

This feeling of being "followers," rather than being in control of their destinies, tends to have a frustrating effect on an educated professional person. Particularly applicable to the baccalaureate degree nurses, this frustration, after having devoted years to training and fine-tuning of skills, translates into a dissatisfaction with the profession. This dissatisfaction is further translated into a high "drop out" rate from the profession.

In some areas of the country, nurses are leaving at a faster rate than replacements can be recruited, creating a major crisis in nursing care. One of the surest methods to reverse this trend, according to those administrators who have tried it, is to increase the participation of the entire nursing staff in vital policy-making decisions.

From the administrative viewpoint, your major concern should be focused on the end results of any proposed program coming from the nursing staff, not necessarily on the individual particulars of the program. To meet the criteria of acceptability, nurse-initiated programs should meet the following four points:

(1) Plan must be in writing, with consent being obtained from the nursing director.
(2) Plan must meet or exceed current standards for quality assurance.
(3) Plan must stay within current budget.
(4) Plan must include evaluation data and a mechanism for program evaluation decisions while it is in progress.

If these four points are met by any nurse-initiated program, you can probably feel fairly comfortable in permitting its initiation within your hospital. The important point to remember is that the trust you display in the nursing staff will enhance their feelings of professionalism, making them feel more valuable to the general management scheme of your hospital.

The results of this change in administrative thinking have been fairly encouraging. Hospitals which have implemented programs of this type have noticed a sizable decline in their nurse departure rate. To illustrate the results further, let's take a look at an actual case where the idea was used.

CASE IN POINT: NURSE-INITIATED PROGRAMMING HELPS ONE MIDWESTERN HOSPITAL CUT ITS NURSE TURNOVER RATE BY OVER 80 PERCENT

For one midwestern hospital, the problem of departing nurses had reached crisis proportions. With an average of 15 percent leaving the hospital's service in one year or less and the rate exceeding 30 percent within two years, the hospital's administration could easily see the need for dramatic changes in policy direction.

After studying the patterns of nurse departures as they correlated with hospital activities, they discovered that resignations declined markedly during any periods when changes were being implemented in the nursing program. This discovery became the *key* to reversing the hospital's problems.

Working in conjunction with the nursing staff, a program of staff participation and openness to change was implemented. The results were very positive toward the goal of nurse retention. Their previous resignation rate, exceeding 30 percent for two years or less, was cut to a 5 percent level after only 2½ years of the program's existence.

With the results of this program, this hospital and others that have utilized it have gained some additional benefits. First, they have been able to make major cuts in the funding for nurse recruiting programs, freeing these funds to be used elsewhere within the hospital. Second, the continuity of operations has been enhanced due to the reduced need for new nurse orientation and the familiarity which is gained by prolonged employment at one facility.

These two factors alone can make a major contribution to the efficiency of any nursing department. By some estimates, staff stability that exceeds three years can represent as much as a 20 percent increase in total efficiency.

(2) Nurse Internship Program

Another innovative program which is being utilized by progressive hospitals, particularly those which actively recruit ex-nurses to return to hospital service, is the Nurse Internship Program.

The basic premise behind this program is to enable the nurse entering the hospital's routine to be "eased into" the daily flow of operations. According to one nursing director who implements this type of program, it permits the incoming nurse to "find her own level," and determine her capabilities and her ultimate patient quantity capacity in actual clinical conditions.

Under this plan, the nurse, whether a recent graduate of a nursing school or a recruited returnee, is first given a brief orientation period, stressing the fundamentals of nursing as they are applied within the individual hospital. Reviews of hospital policy are conducted and discussions of the individual's job expectations in the classroom setting are encouraged.

After the classroom portion of the program is completed, the nurse is brought on duty for the hospital, being given responsibility for one or two patients at the initial stage. As the nurse becomes further acclimated to the hospital's routine, this patient number is gradually increased to the full load normally expected of all other nurses employed by the hospital.

By abandoning the old "sink or swim" ethic of hurling the full load immediately onto a new nurse, the initial fears of failure, which cause the greatest number of early resignations, are eliminated.

In terms of tangible results, the nurse internship program has proven to be quite effective, particularly if it is teamed up with an ongoing orientation and general training program. By uniting these programs, you can effectively limit the administrative overhead of implementing the program in addition to improving the internship's coordination with the director's general objectives for the nursing program.

To underscore the internship program's success in combating the rising tide of nursing resignations, let's examine the results which were obtained by one hospital that initiated this type of program.

CASE IN POINT: MICHIGAN HOSPITAL'S NURSE INTERNSHIP PROGRAM CUTS TURNOVER RATE DRAMATICALLY

In an effort to combat the dual problems of nursing staff turnover and shortfalls in recruiting goals, one hospital in northern Michigan decided to implement an ongoing nurse internship program for its hospital. Using a combined class for both new nursing school graduates and those nurses wishing to re-enter the clinical care arena, the hospital began to make major strides in the areas of staff recruitment and retention.

From a point of virtual crisis caused by nurse resignations, the nurse internship program was able to cut the turnover rate by 30 percent within one year of the program's implementation. This trend is expected to continue even further as the program's total impact is felt within the hospital.

According to nursing directors who are familiar with the system, the single greatest benefit of this program is the non-pressurized atmosphere that is created for new nurses joining the hospital's staff. By maintaining a positive working experience, particularly in the early period of her employment, the ultimate contribution of the nurse to total staff performance will be considerably better.

"Confidence," stated one nursing director, "is the key factor in the program. If we can instill confidence in the nurse's mind when she joins our health care team, her self-image and her professionalism on the job will be enhanced to such a degree as to eliminate most of the need for continuous supervisory surveillance. The professionalism will be automatic, not 'force-fed' by the fear of dismissal."

Procedural Manuals: "Bibles" of Administrative Policy

From the administrative standpoint, the single greatest issue regarding the nursing staff's functions is the effective translation of hospital policy into daily action. The common vehicle for this translation is the "Nursing Procedural Manual."

Commonly referred to by the above name or, in some cases, as the "Nursing Policy Manual," the book's intent is to maintain consistent interpretation of hospital policy and procedure, placing the required activities of the nursing staff into written form.

To simplify the reference process, let's briefly review the essential elements which should be included in every hospital's Nursing Procedural Manual.

Elements of the Manual

(1) Define "chain of command" positions and their relationships in hospital operations.

(2) Define individual nurse responsibilities.

(3) General organizational information.

(4) Departmental functions and limitations.

(5) Clearly define all policies regarding employment.

(6) Establish staffing patterns for 24-hour nursing service coverage.

(7) State policies on professional and nonprofessional private practice nurses to augment regular nursing staff.

(8) Delineate the roles of volunteers, including patients' family members, in any nursing activities.

(9) State hospital policy on standard in-service training, including minimum standards.

(10) Cover legal aspects; i.e., witnessing of wills, signatures, agreements or marriages for patients.

(11) Rules for requisition, care, and use of all nursing equipment and supplies.

(12) Hospital policy for public relations and the release of information to employees, public, and the press.

(13) Written standards for maintenance of nursing care units and related facilities.

(14) Safety rules and reporting procedures. (It is advisable to give emphasis to hazards of smoking in certain areas, particularly as applicable to anesthesia, oxygen, and therapy gas treatments, as applicable in inhalation therapy cases.)

(15) Define nursing department responsibilities in preparation for, and during, disasters.

(16) Policies for effective coordination with the housekeeping and food service departments.

(17) Standards for nursing records and reports.

(18) Detailed policy on patient admission procedures.

(19) Name staff member or members authorized to receive and implement the written, verbal, telephoned, and standing orders issued by members of the medical staff.

(20) Establish daily routines for patient care, including details on procedures.

(21) Crisis care management, including procedures for shock, hemorrhage, the critically ill, with policy on reporting to physicians, family, clergy, and the business office.

(22) Communicable disease management procedures, including isolation techniques and hazards which contribute to hospital-induced infections.

(23) Medication control procedures, with emphasis on narcotics, poisons, hypnotics, and all radioactive substances.

(24) Policy on using patient restraints.

(25) Reporting procedures for missing patients.

(26) Control procedures for food and medications brought to hospital by patients and/or visitors.

(27) Control and disposal of unused medicines.

(28) Responsibilities for health education and information dissemination for patients.

(29) Patient transfers between departments.

(30) Nursing policy toward, and cooperation with, the clergy and patients' religious activities.

(31) Visiting hours, rules for visitor control, and policy implementation for children's visits.

(32) Patient discharge procedures and attendant notification requirements.

(33) Required procedures for release against medical advice.

(34) Established procedures following a patient's death; i.e., moving of remains, notification of family, etc.

The preceding elements, if provided in a properly integrated text, will provide adequate safeguards to be certain that the administrative policies of your hospital will be consistently implemented. From your viewpoint, this consistency must be considered as the number one priority of administrative objective. Without this necessary consistency, the potential for severe problems in medical procedures and public relations matters could prove to be a major source of problems and concern in the future.

The Nursing Service: Some Final Thoughts

Throughout this chapter, the emphasis has been on the procedural aspects of nursing department operations. One vital element, however, has not been discussed. Yet, its importance to the ultimate success of the clinical mission is unsurpassed. Without *compassion* for the patients she helps, the most procedurally proficient nurse will be little more than a dispensing machine for medications.

Compassion, the quality that can never be taught, must come from within every successful nurse. The sense of security instilled by a nurse who cares can often make the difference between recovery and lingering illness or, in the worst cases, even death. It is the ultimate healing agent that can't be dispensed with a pill or injected with a hypodermic needle.

While our emphasis should continue to be on the elements which contribute to nursing department efficiency, we should never lose sight of, or seek to sacrifice, the "compassion factor" in the interests of maximum productivity standards. The hospital is a very special place, having its unique set of psychological requirements which must be met.

The well-trained compassionate nurse has the "tools" to meet this objective, easing both the physical and psychological sufferings of the patients she serves. With a small measure of administrative restraint, these "Angels of Mercy" can be free to fulfill this special mission for your hospital and the patients it serves. *

---

* See also ¶4101 *et seq.,* Prentice-Hall *Hospital Cost Management Service.*

How to maintain and enhance efficiency in laboratory services

13

FROM THE DAY WHEN PHYSICIANS PRACTICED MEDICINE strictly from the black bag they carried, basing their diagnostic prowess on past experience and a prayer for luck, to the advanced diagnostic mechanism that operates today, the contrast is startling. As one of the fundamental parts of today's diagnostic process, the hospital lab service plays an integral role in the quality of health care being delivered.

In this chapter, we will review some of the essential elements of operating an efficient and effective hospital laboratory and clinical pathology department. The interrelationship between these two similar, yet distinguishably different, services provides a clear picture of the scope and advanced capabilities of this area of medicine.

Defining "Clinical Lab"

Clinical laboratory services, in the strictest definition, contain the elements of bacteriology, hematology, serology, urinalysis, etc. To "laymanize" this, we would state that Clinical Lab is the "Fluid Science" portion of the laboratory's activities.

Within this context, based on current technology, approximately 90 different tests could be prescribed. Yet, in routine daily operation, fewer than a dozen different tests are actually performed. This relatively small variety comprises over 60 percent of the workload involved in the lab.

Defining "Clinical Pathology"

By contrast, clinical pathology is most often associated with the study of solid tissue structures of the human body. This function ranges from the examination of tissue removed during surgical procedures to performing autopsies in determining "Cause of Death."

In addition to serving as a double-check system for the performance of the hospital's medical and surgical staffs, the hospital pathologist also serves a vital role in the area of criminal justice. In some areas, the pathologist also doubles as the city or county coroner.

Acting in the role of Coroner or Medical Examiner (interchangable terms to reflect the same role), the pathologist helps to judge whether or not an individual's death was the result of "natural causes" or came from injuries of a criminally-based nature. The judgments of the coroner have major effects on criminal court proceedings, insurance benefits to beneficiaries, and a host of other areas. The pathologist, even more than other members of the med staff, plays *the* prominent role in the public's perception of medicine's "Quality Control."

Departmental Organization

Essentially, the power structure of the laboratory centers around the clinical pathologist. The pathologist must be a competent physician with specific background in pathological studies, preferably eligible for board certification by the American Board of Pathology.

Directly under the pathologist, a group of medical technologists translate the expertise of the pathologist into the effective operations of the laboratory. These technologists must also meet certain minimum standards of qualification, sufficient to be eligible for the Registry of Medical Technologists. This registry is under the sponsorship of the American Society of Clinical Pathologists.

The medical technologists, in addition to performing most of the testing and the "hands on" work of the lab, are responsible for supervising the laboratory assistants who perform the incidental chores which assure smooth laboratory management and performance.

Variable Layout Planning: An Essential Element

The physical layout of the laboratory facilities is probably the largest contributing factor to overall efficiency. One of the greatest dangers in lab planning is to "lock in" laboratory facilities to a fixed technological level, leaving no room to develop services to meet expanded hospital needs and advancements in equipment technology.

For this reason, choice of a lab's location must include provisions for possible expansion of its floor plan. Each portion of a lab's activities must have adequate space provided for permit comfortable performance of the duties involved.

Layout planning must provide adequate space for equipment and personnel for each of three essential areas:

(1) Administrative.
(2) Technical.
(3) Auxiliary.

Each of these three subdivisions has its own specific physical requirements which are designed to meet the needs of efficiency and comfortable working conditions for staff members. To understand the needs of each, let's take a quick review of some basic requirements you should be looking for.

(1) Administrative

The Administrative subdivision should contain five essential elements; a waiting room, a venipuncture cubicle, specimen toilet, basal metabolism-electrocardiography room, and the area specifically set aside as the pathologist's office (a form of private study area).

The waiting room is set up for the convenience of the ambulatory patients visiting the lab. Furnished in the usual fashion for such areas, it includes a desk for the clerk-typist as well as for the pathologist's secretary. A communications system between this area and the technical area, including the pathologist's office, is recommended.

The venipuncture cubical is another feature that is provided for the ambulatory patients referred to the laboratory. Walk-in patients may have blood samples taken here for lab testing.

The specimen toilet is the facility for collecting urine and stool samples. Efficient layout design would place the specimen toilet area adjacent to the technical area, preferrably near the urinalysis unit. A pass window incorporated into the toilet facility would enhance transfer of specimens into the laboratory area.

The basal metabolism-electrocardiography room's purpose is relatively self-explanatory. This area is often also used in conjunction with the hospital's blood bank activities, providing a place to obtain blood from donors. In addition to technical paraphernalia needed for its function, a desk and adjacent lavatory should also be included.

As implied earlier, the pathologist's office itself serves as an "inner sanctum" for the doctor. Separated by a glass partition from the technical area, this would permit the pathologist to observe the working area while reducing noise levels sometimes inherent in a busy lab. This area can be equipped with a draw curtain to provide privacy, particularly during times when distractions might impede some vital aspect of his work.

The office interior should include the standard desk facilities, plus a working table suitable for a microscope and related equipment. This permits the pathologist to study tissue samples in an undisturbed setting.

(2) Technical Area

The technical area incorporates the various testing equipment that every lab facility needs to carry out its mission in the health care picture. Efficiency demands that this area be divided into the various subdivisions, based on the activities required of the lab.

Some of these subdivisions might include Hematology, Biochemistry, Parasitology, Bacteriology, Blood Bank, and Serology.

Each of these subdivisions is commonly referred to as a *unit*. As part of the laboratory design, a *Unitized Design Concept* is employed. Based on the projected needs for each unit, their positions are determined in the layout.

Here's how the Unitized Design Concept works. As mentioned a short while ago, the vital necessity is to avoid being "locked in" on the current lab design. Proper implementation of this design concept would prevent this problem.

The first priority in the design area is to determine the projected unit needs. If a unit is not projected to experience growth, its location is not such a large concern. The only concern is to limit the amount of staff travel time in performing the needed duties.

The major area of concern in lab design is the location of units which are projected to experience major growth. These units should, whenever possible, be located on the outer perimeters of the lab facility. This would limit the extent of any remodeling efforts needed to quickly expand available space in response to the demonstrated needs.

For example, your current blood bank facilities might be perfectly adequate to meet the projected needs of your in-hospital blood use. However, if the blood bank were to be used for the needs of the Public Health Service, its size might be woefully inadequate to meet the demand. If no design provisions are made for expansion, you might be locked out from an excellent revenue-producing option in the future.

Laboratory management flexibility could be enhanced by utilizing movable partitions, particularly in areas where their use would not compromise the quality of lab performance. Essentially, the movable partitions would permit space requirements to be adjusted as the needs of individual units would indicate.

Due to the infinitely possible variables involved in lab management, no solid guidelines on lab size can be reliably formulated. Conventional wisdom has placed minimum lab size at one square foot per 25 lab tests annually. Hence, using this formula, a lab that runs 25,000 tests annually requires 1,000 square feet of laboratory space.

The most important design consideration is to make the lab a comfortable and efficient place for its staff. In addition to providing enhanced productivity, these considerations also play an important role in recruiting new laboratory staff members. An attractive work area will enhance your hospital's list of qualified applicants for the available positions.

(3) Auxiliary Area

Commonly located adjacent to both administrative and technical areas, the Auxiliary Service section serves many of the peripheral activities commonly associated with hospital laboratory functions. The variety of services involved in auxiliary units depends directly on the requirements of the individual lab.

All laboratories require a glasswashing and sterilization unit or units, preferably centrally located to the areas of heaviest demand. Most often, this would be adjacent to serology, bacteriology, and biochemistry units. Separate doors directly from these units to the sterilizing room are advisable, preventing accidental contamination of other laboratory testing procedures.

Each sterilizing room requires, at minimum, a water still, sterilizing oven, pressure sterilizer, and a pipette washer. Due to the heat generated by these equipment items, adequate ventilation must be provided to insure employee comfort.

Laboratories which utilize test animals for their work must have an auxiliary unit to care for the animals, separate facilities for their testing, and adequate sanitation provisions for the animals' quarters.

The hospital morgue, necroscopy, and specimen storage areas, usually located in the hospital's basement, are included in the auxiliary service planning for the laboratory. Though located away from the traffic areas for patients and visitors, they should nonetheless be within easy access to elevators to promote efficiency.

Depending on the size and general mission of your hospital, the pathology department may also incorporate such areas as clinical photography, medical illustration, research, and related functions into its program. This would be particularly true if your hospital were affiliated with medical education. Expanding the boundaries of available knowledge and offering opportunities for more varied experiences to students would make these functions a particularly valuable adjunct to the educational process.

Dynamics of Expanded Service

During times when almost everyone involved in hospital administration is looking for ways to slash overhead to stabilize costs, raising the subject of expanding laboratory services might seem hypocritical. Surprisingly, there is clear evidence that expansion of available services and major reductions in outlay for hospital lab facilities *can be accomplished concurrently*.

The key to this idea is to incorporate laboratory functions from two hospitals, preferably located near each other, to eliminate duplication of services. The lab tests performed at one facility would not be performed at the other. The same concept of cooperation, though on a considerably smaller scale, could be done with a small diagnostic clinic which refers patients to your hospital.

In all too many cases, there is competition, rather than cooperation, for the business generated by such routine lab tests as urinalysis. If both facilities are performing a particular test, consolidation of these functions would seem to be the route to go.

Thanks to advances in computer science, transmission of information between two facilities would not represent an impediment to the program. The interconnection would actually represent an added feature to enhance efficiency.

Through cooperation, the combined productivity of two lab facilities could be more than doubled in a relatively short time. Though this system does have a few potential problem spots (transfer of specimens between facilities, billing responsibility, etc.), these minor problems can be easily and productively circumvented.

To illustrate this idea, let's take a closer look at two facilities which implemented this idea of enhanced productivity.

CASE IN POINT: COMBINED LAB COORDINATION BOOSTS TOTAL PRODUCTIVITY BY OVER 120 PERCENT

In an effort to limit costs and enhance the levels of service available to patients, two midwestern hospitals, one a Veterans' Administration facility and the other a Medical Center, decided to coordinate their laboratory functions.

Basing their division of responsibility on which facility had the more sophisticated equipment, the V.A. facility was designated to run the less complex laboratory tests. The Medical Center was then able to concentrate its laboratory's attention on the more complex testing procedures for which it was so admirably equipped.

As an initial benefit, both facilities found that their "per procedure" laboratory space requirements were slashed by 30 percent. Because of this fact, both facilities were able to offer a larger variety of available tests and increase the precision of their diagnostic procedures to a marked degree.

As the primary benefit, the increased specialization of lab functions permitted far greater productivity by reducing mobility of staff members within the facility. Staff members could remain at their stations and run a whole string of similar tests with the same equipment, making them operate at a level closer to their designed capacity. This also improved staff morale by permitting lab assistants and technologists to specialize in tests with which they felt most proficient.

In a study of results after four years, the productivity improvements were phenomenal. The total number of tests performed annually by the two facilities jumped by almost 125 percent.

With the inclusion of interconnected computers, feeding results from one facility to the other was simplified, marking a major improvement in procedures from what was used when both labs operated in the "solo" mode. The billing problem was solved by having tests billed from the facility from which the tested specimens originated.

The above illustration clearly shows the positive benefits of consolidating services. About the only place in which this system would *not* be advisable is in cases where facilities are so far apart as to make specimen transfers impractical.

When the additional revenues generated by rising productivity enter the picture, investment in new and even more efficient equipment can become a practical reality. This pyramiding of results means that the preliminary improvements shown by the consolidation program may be only the beginning. One good improvement helps to build further improvements.

In the final analysis, the concept of laboratory service consolidation may be just the right ticket for a financially pressed hospital. The end result of the program is to enable the lab service to provide larger variety and better overall quality without adding enormously to the total costs.

Public Insurance and the Laboratory Crisis

As a constantly growing segment of our society joins the ranks of Senior Citizens, the role of our public health reimbursement system (Medicare, Medicaid, etc.) continues to grow. This fact represents another factor in the availability of funding to support vitally needed services.

Politicians in Washington and in various state capitals, often well-meaning but sometimes misguided (if you listen to people having to wade through bureaucratic paperwork), have evolved a complex system that forces gross inefficiencies on laboratory services. As one pathologist put it, "We spend almost as much time filling out forms to comply with government regulations as we do to perform the work which necessitates the forms."

Though public reimbursement agencies do not represent the only source for this problem, they undoubtedly play a major role in creating it. But the greatest problem is in the area of reimbursement amounts and their timing. Late and sometimes inadequate payments can quickly create major cash flow problems.

This fact makes effective cost control systems for the hospital laboratory a virtual necessity. Considering the fact that 30 to 50 percent (more in some hospitals) of lab revenue comes from these sources, restrictions in increases or even reductions in some cases can have a major detrimental impact on the quality of a hospital's lab service.

As this problem has increased, a new trend toward rejecting direct reimbursement has been instituted by some hospitals. Theoretically, the system's idea makes the patient financially liable for services rendered, removing the controls which reimbursement agencies would seek to impose on laboratory and general hospital operations.

Though the concept appears superficially attractive, serious problems can result from this system which could be larger than those created by direct reimbursement. As an example, the extent of charges may be large enough to make the patient unable to pay. Second, there is no guarantee that the patient will pay *any* of the money owed for services. If the patient spends the reimbursement money for something else, the hospital and its lab could get stuck with a major financial loss.

Where does this leave the laboratory management picture? With either payment method, a substantial "gray" area in the legal picture exists. As government agencies seek to restrict their payments, there remains a question of fee limits. Can a lab, for example, charge the patient for amounts which are not approved by Medicare or Medicaid?

Though an ever-increasing number of Medicare beneficiaries have also purchased supplementary coverage from private insurance firms, these companies will usually honor only the amounts *approved by Medicare* as the legitimate amount for claims against them.

The concept of justifiable cost is also a cornerstone of state Medicaid-type programs. Quite often, there is a substantial disparity between what these programs view as justifiable and the opinion of the hospital. In most cases, the difference between the standard fees and amounts approved is never made up from any sources.

Financial shortfalls created by this problem would, in some cases, be made up by altered fee schedules for patients not under the restrictive structure of state or federal programs. But here, again, the specter of the private insurance industry throws a logjam into the scenario.

Many private insurers also operate under the policy of "approved" rates for hospital services. If a hospital accepts direct reimbursement, particularly if no prior understanding is made concerning coverage shortfalls, there may be no legal way to collect the remaining balance of fees owed.

When you trace this rather confusing picture to its completion, you come back to the one saving premise which we mentioned earlier—cost containment. In some, if not a majority of, cases, a hospital may be able to get adequate reimbursement for services if an active effort at cost containment can be proven to the insurance carriers. If you can prove that your hospital is providing services at the lowest prices possible under the present conditions of your facilities, you are quite likely to receive almost all of the money to which you claim entitlement.

For the lab, this means a record of suspected conditions for which tests were ordered, findings of the tests, and the ultimate diagnosis which was made possible by laborary analysis. Though the amount of detail for these records can prove somewhat time-consuming, the records can often spell the difference between an acceptable payment and a rotten deal.

Forms and Records

The variety of your laboratory's forms will, to a large extent, be determined by the number of services which are provided. For efficiency, keeping form numbers to a minimum would be advisable. With the added consideration of total printing costs, this advisory is one which helps to maintain course on the cost containment objective.

The most common forms encountered in the lab are lumped together under the heading, *Procedure Request Forms*. These forms, often consolidated into one unit, are often found in a multi-copy format. This helps to avoid repetition in processing lab tests information at the business office, within the lab, and to the prescribing physician. When one form achieves these multiple objectives simultaneously, enhanced efficiency is always the final product.

The basic purpose of the procedure request forms is to maintain records of lab test requests, including date of request, date performed, and recording of the results obtained. By having all information available on one form, the potential for major record-keeping foul-ups is virtually eliminated.

In some cases, such as blood sugar analysis and basal metabolism tests, these requests must be made a minimum of one day in advance. This permits the patient to make appropriate preparations for the test, helping to assure the accurary of results. This same principle would apply to electrocardiography procedures.

For the purposes of long-term record-keeping procedures, the centrally important format is the Daily Record Ledger. This serves as a double-check mechanism for levels of laboratory activity on a monthly and annual basis. By checking these figures periodically with those in the accounting department, the business office can be reasonably certain of having its procedures accurate and collecting adequate fees to compensate for lab tests performed. These daily ledgers can be purchased in stock printed form, helping to limit costs.

Special Economy Note: Depending on your lab's activity level, you might find it economical to buy ledgers in slightly larger quantities, cutting their per unit cost.

For the functions of the clinical pathology section, the major additional form to be considered is the consent form for autopsy. Though some hospitals may rely on a verbal consent, most legal analysts agree that a hospital is on much firmer legal ground by obtaining written approval from the next of kin or legal guardian of the remains. This written consent should also include the permission to retain diseased tissue or organs for further laboratory examination.

The area of obtaining this approval can be the most challenging of any aspect of pathology department activity. Balancing the need for further medical knowledge against the psychological needs of survivors undergoing the enormous stresses entailed by death, gentle tact and diplomacy are the order of the day. In some cases, the task may be best delegated to the family's religious advisor, often present in these cases. In any event, the time factor is of paramount importance. Promptness in performing autopsies helps to assure the accuracy of the results obtained.

The autopsy also generates paper work going to people and agencies outside of the hospital. The Death Certificate is a prime example of such paper work. This is usually presented to the next of kin, serving as the legal proof of death for estate and other purposes.

Further, there is the detailed report of the results of the autopsy. This report is filed with the pathologist's records, with copies going to Medical Records and to the attending physician for the deceased patient.

These reports are also referred to regular meetings of the applicable physicians' committee. Often somewhat euphemistically referred to as "The Death Committee," the routine Mortality Conference studies all available data on each death in a hospital, trying to discover if it was preventable, and attempting to discern if there are methods to avoid a recurrence in the future.

Closing Thoughts on Lab Management

As the reliance of diagnostic medicine turns in increasing amounts to the hospital lab, along with its greater impact on the total bill paid by patients, the pressures for effective cost controls on lab activities will increase. There is no real way to avoid this problem. The pathology department will unavoidably become subject to these pressures.

The best way to reduce the potential problems is to initiate firm cost controls into your pathology program now, if they are not in place already. These should include statistics on per test costs, supply usage controls, strict monitoring of waste, and detailed inventory procedures to be certain that your other procedures are gaining the desired results.

Thanks to the large variety of items involved, the best route for monitoring these functions is through the use of a small computer. The running totals which these computers can maintain will give the department's chief the most current information possible. This enables the pathologist to quickly ascertain areas where waste is occurring and stop it before the results prove very detrimental to the department's budget.

Perhaps the best way to illustrate this is to review the case of one western state's hospital using a computer for this purpose.

CASE IN POINT: COMPUTER-MONITORED HOSPITAL LAB CUTS COSTS BY MAJOR AMOUNT

For one hospital's pathology department in the western U.S., the specter of waste forced a time of reckoning for the hospital's department chief and its administrator. Permitted to continue indefinitely, the waste was slated to siphon off several thousands of dollars from the department's effective working budget annually.

With the installation of a new minicomputer to keep a running calculation of inventories and expenses, the department was able to slash at least 15 percent from its supply costs by pinpointing the major areas of avoidable waste in lab operations.

Due to the size of the department's annual supply budget, the elimination of waste paid for the computer system in slightly over a year, making all further savings generated by the system "pure gravy" for the hospital's profit outlook.

The above case study clearly proves that effective cost control can be accomplished. The information which has been provided in this chapter should be considered as only a springboard for further ideas and experimentation within the department. New ideas and concepts that further advance the cause of cost control are being developed even as you read these words.

But, despite this emphasis on cost control, the ultimate criterion for departmental success is the level of quality which can be maintained for pathology department performance. Without this quality emphasis, any other discussion is purely academic. We must never sacrifice this vital element in the zeal to "keep the lid on" the laboratory's price tag for operations.

Dedicated personnel and some common sense in your approach will yield major results, assuring that your hospital's lab will offer the best possible services that your facility's financial resources and incoming revenue will permit. *

---

* See also ¶5401 *et seq.,* Prentice-Hall *Hospital Cost Service Management.*

The key elements for effective and efficient radiology services 14

WITH TECHNOLOGICAL ADVANCES OCCURRING AT A DAZ-ZLING RATE, the x-ray department of today and that of only ten years ago can be worlds apart. The new engineering advances have resulted in new uses for the x-ray, plus modified application techniques which reduce hazards. This reduced hazard level makes its expanded utilization a feasible though costly application of radiology's future rule.

Here, as in other areas of hospital management, the expanded technology has increased the challenges to fundamental management concepts. New technology has a price tag. This cost must be weighed with the projected benefits, along with the price that health care consumers are willing and able to pay.

This dual challenge is the essence of radiology's future. Steering a prudent course, potentially a conservative one, is becoming a necessity of today's social climate.

Meeting this challenge requires that the department is competently organized, has adequate facilities and equipment to fulfill its role within the hospital's management scheme, and maintains its efficiency in daily operation. If these divergent elements are executed simultaneously, the end result will be an effective and efficient radiology department.

Departmental Organization

At the head of the radiology department is the staff radiologist, a graduate of a recognized medical school with additional training in the specialty of radiology. Though not mandatory, most hospitals prefer their staff radiologist to be a Diplomate of the American Board of Radiology.

Directly beneath the radiologist on the organizational ladder are the x-ray technologists. Their function is to perform the work of the department, under the

171

direct supervision of the radiologist. The use of x-ray diagnostic procedures and other departmental functions dictate that three to five technologists per hundred beds of hospital capacity are employed in the radiology department.

The relationship of the radiologist with other aspects of the hospital's authority structure, though usually determined by official hospital policy, makes him responsible first to the medical staff structure for clinical activities. All matters involving departmental administration, the business aspects, come under the administrator's jurisdiction.

The basic points of interconnection between the radiology department and other hospital subdivisions are with the medical staff, the patient care units, outpatient department, and the business office.

The business office has a direct effect on the profitability, or lack thereof, of the radiology department because of its role in handling the charge slips and assisting in determining the price schedule for all radiological examinations.

Departmental Facilities

One of the greatest difficulties in assessing the facility requirements of the hospital radiology department is making adequate allowances for technological advances in the field. Standard x-ray equipment which has been the measure of excellence for radiology has been augmented by sound-wave technology and scanner computerized diagnostic equipment.

This last development, scanner technology, has served to reduce the need for exploratory surgery and effectively expanded the range of radiological services which hospitals can provide. This major advance has also increased the space requirements of the department by a substantial degree.

While these newest developments are, at the time of this writing, still too costly to be considered by smaller hospitals, a declining trend in computer technology prices should make these current advances available and financially feasible by the end of the 1980's.

This factor makes it imperative to plan potential expansion capabilities into any current planning structures for the department. Demands for radiology services have historically doubled every ten years. This demand may be accelerated by double-checks which some potentially "gun shy" physicians might require to assure maximum safety from malpractice litigation.

In addition to this, requirements for documentation by federal and state agencies plus minimum standards set by the Joint Commission on the Accreditation of Hospitals continue to accelerate the demands made on radiological equipment and facilities.

The primary role played by radiological services in the diagnostic process makes their requirements a prime concern during any development planning done for construction or remodeling of the hospital. In the majority of cases, the radiologist is called in to consult on design changes which affect diagnostic procedures.

Specific design requirements for department facilities begin by dividing the total available space into the four basic sections for effective operations; (1) the waiting room, (2) radiologist's office and viewing rooms (sometimes combined into one unit), (3) the radiographic room, and (4) darkroom facilities.

While the individual space needs vary with the nature of hospital functions, the common standards indicate a range of between 20 and 50 square feet of radiology department space per hospital bed. The absolute minimum to be considered would be 400 to 600 square feet, even for the smallest of hospitals today.

The total space requirements are determined by a considerable number of factors. In addition to the common demands for inpatient, emergency, and outpatient services, allowances should be made for activity generated by outside clinics, private physicians, employee and student health programs, health department activities, and any projected shared-service agreements which might be initiated with other hospitals.

To firmly outline general departmental requirements, let's take a brief overview of the four sections of the department's facilities mentioned a short while ago.

(1) The Waiting Room

If the radiology department is run on a reasonably efficient schedule, there is no major need for waiting room facilities. A reasonable space should be provided (sufficient to avoid additional patient anxiety due to cramped conditions) with a few chairs available for comfortable seating. Under normal circumstances, patients would not be required to spend much time here.

(2) The Radiologist's Office and Viewing Room

In terms of general requirements, the radiologist's office does not represent substantially different requirements from other professionals housed within the hospital. Aside from the standard office furnishings, the needs of the office can be modified when the office and viewing room are one combined facility.

In the combined setup, the specially lighted x-ray viewer is also included into the office's scheme, often being a hanging wall model sufficiently large to accommodate the largest x-ray films.

The overall size of the radiologist's office is generally determined by the activity level of the department as well as by the personal preferences of the resident radiologist.

(3) The Radiographic Room

As the main staging area for the department's daily activities, the radiographic room also presents the most detailed and precise requirements of any rooms involved in the department's work. Due to the special safety considerations involved in the use of x-ray equipment, the location of the room and its construction features are of paramount importance.

Due to the special costs involved in construction, locating the room on an outside wall is the first major step in limiting the price tag. Due to the high cost of the lead wall coating, necessary to restrict the spread of x-ray radiation, the outside wall location reduces the cost by eliminating the need for one wall's coating.

The entrance to the radiographic room must be wide enough to permit easy entry for wheelchair or stretcher cases. The usual standard for door width has been recognized as between 3 feet 10 inches and a full 4 feet. This can be varied somewhat to cut costs, going with the standard manufactured doors (rather than custom-built), as long as the smaller figure previously mentioned is used as the minimum standard.

The interior of the room must also be designed to accommodate the specialized needs presented by the non-ambulatory entrants, giving sufficient room to effect easy transfers from wheelchairs or stretchers. Most references place the minimum at 12 feet by 18 feet. Here, again, this standard can be modified upward, depending on the amount and nature of the department's activities.

Fixtures for the room, aside from standard equipment for radiographic activities, should definitely include a sink and toilet within easy access. Because fluoroscopy is also performed here, lightproof shades should also be included for the room.

While centralization of the department's activities is considered a worthwhile objective from the efficiency standpoint, the specialized needs of a hospital's surgical team may require that x-ray examinations of fractures and cystoscopic exams commonly conducted by the radiology department be done in facilities very near to the operating rooms.

If departmental centralization must become the overriding concern, the best route to follow is to place the entire radiology department's facilities as near to the surgical suites as can be practically accomplished.

(4) The Darkroom

The general design of the radiographic darkroom requires that sufficient space is available for the needed darkroom equipment and a lightproof entrance is provided. Though some differences of opinion exist on the best type of entrance, the locked door with a gasketed edge to seal out light seems to be the major preference.

Another desirable feature which helps to minimize or eliminate x-ray film damage is a film transfer cabinet, making the transfer of film from the radiographic room to the darkroom safer and more efficient. However, for the best interests of the department, the nature of the equipment and room layout should be left to the radiologist and the manufacturing engineer.

The layout and conditions of the interior of the darkroom are equally important as they pertain to operator comfort and the successful handling of x-ray materials. Temperatures within the room should be maintained at 72 degrees F., with a humidity reading at 50 percent. Ventilation statistics should measure the air flow at ten feet per second.

The room must contain both standard and safe light features, with wall coloration permitting maximum reflection of the safe light illumination. Wiring for the room must be made to conform to local codes as well as those standards set by the

National Board of Fire Underwriters. Whenever possible, the power supply for the radiology department should be on its own separate circuit, preventing the possibility of disastrous voltage variations.

Computers Changing the Scene

With the development of new high-speed technologies for increased efficiency, the look of modern radiology is beginning a period of rapid change. Some experts believe that the x-ray department of the late 1980's will be as radically different as the changes effected between 1960 and 1980.

The increased utilization of computer technology, along with its continuing decline in cost, has opened the door to major improvements in efficiency for the field of radiology. Computer-programmed precision settings of x-ray equipment are beginning to take away the margin of human error, improving the efficiency and accuracy of radiographic work.

The marriage of ultrasound technology and the computer revolution has presented new, challenging uses for radiological services, making them an increasingly valuable ally in the science and art of surgery. To underscore the importance of this alliance with the computer, let's take a look at a case where it's being utilized.

CASE IN POINT: COMPUTER TECHNOLOGY CUTS RADIOGRAPHIC EXAM AND INTERPRETATION TIME BY OVER EIGHTY PERCENT

Faced with an increasing demand for x-ray services, but reluctant to add staff and standard radiographic equipment to its department, one midwestern hospital began examining the possibility of letting a computer assist the x-ray process.

"We knew that major improvements in efficiency were required to meet the increased demand for radiological services," the hospital's chief of radiology stated. "Thanks to this computer, we've been able to reduce the time between exposure to the readable x-ray image from minutes to a matter of seconds."

The system he was talking about translates the x-ray picture taken into a visual image which is shown on a viewing screen. All of this happens while the permanent film, designed to be stored for the patient's medical records is being processed. In addition, with the press of a single button, an extra print can be made for review by the attending physician.

As an end result, the capacity of the hospital's x-ray department has more than doubled, making the proposed addition to departmental staff unnecessary. The total efficiency, thanks to this new equipment, was enhanced by an estimated 82 percent.

This single case dramatically illustrates the tremendous power and potential of computer technology. The only negative element, already mentioned in discussions for computers in other chapters, is the matter of cost. The real key to deciding on computerization is the level of projected use that the equipment will have.

Standard Radiology Policies

In similar fashion to other hospital departments, the radiology department must have a specific set of policies for its operations, written and recorded with the hospital's administrative offices to maintain consistency of implementation. Though these policies may vary somewhat from one hospital to another, the following list of general policy objectives has been followed by most radiology departments. Some of the policy elements are dictated by state and/or federal regulations, precluding variations.

Policies for a Radiology Department

(1) Radiology department services must be made available to meet the needs of good patient care according to currently recognized standards of medical and radiological practice.

(2) The radiologist must have an established schedule for attendance in the department, sufficient to conduct examinations, x-ray readings, any pre-scribed treatments, and consultations with medical staff members, as required.

(3) Total responsibility for all departmental activities rests with the radiologist.

(4) According to the standards of the Joint Commission on Hospital Accreditation, the department must retain the services of one registered technologist, with responsibilities to take and process x-ray films. The technologist is, however, prohibited from interpretation or consultation functions for the department.

(5) The radiologist is to be a consulting member of the hospital's medical staff, subject to the benefits and restrictions that such membership implies.

(6) All radiologic reports from the department must be signed by the radiologist.

(7) All reports and x-ray films must be made available to the referring physician.

(8) All films remain the property of the hospital.

(9) Any films or reports compiled by the department are part of the patient's medical record, subject to the same rules imposed on records generated by other hospital departments.

(10) In compliance with legal requirements, films must be retained for a minimum period of five to seven years for clinical reference or medico-legal considerations. Films which represent value for research can be retained indefinitely.

(11) All films must be legibly and permanently marked for reference purposes.

(12) Established safety rules are to be incorporated into the written policy for the department.

(13) Established procedures must be maintained for proper aseptic technique, with special emphasis on the disposal of infectious materials.

(14) If permitted in the operating room, x-ray equipment must have special provisions to limit electrostatic accumulation. These controls must conform to the standards of the National Fire Protective Association.

(15) All department employees must be subject to complete annual physicals, with blood counts taken every six months from employees who face routine radiation exposure.

(16) Provisions must be made to maintain accurate radiologic records for clinical and administrative use.

(17) Rules for the control and use of radioactive materials must adhere to the standards set by the United States Atomic Energy Commission.

Liability Insurance: Safety Cuts the Cost

Aside from the obvious health benefits which proper safety procedures bring to departmental employees, the hospital can also enjoy a substantial cost benefit in special considerations offered by some insurance carriers. Depending on the company involved, liability rates can be cut by substantial amounts, based on lengths of time without claimable injuries or losses, safety rules implemented by the department, or other considerations. By emphasizing the safety angle so extensively, the insurance companies enjoy substantial benefits. In passing along some of the fruits of safety-conscious operations, they encourage closer adherence to standards. On the long term, this presents an even greater savings to the insurance carriers.

To exploit this safety-insurance rate connection to its maximum, you might find it advisable to check your current policies for any tie-in between rates and your safety record and/or procedures. If your current policy does not offer this type of benefit, you might consider shopping around for another insurance company. You might find, as a number of other hospitals have, that your insurance rates could drop by as much as 25 percent.

Radiology—Some Trends in the Wind

While we do not pretend to have an infallible crystal ball before our eyes, some new and potentially exciting trends in the area of radiology are on the horizon. These trends could completely revolutionize the methods and scope of radiological services as we know them today.

The continuing advance of computer technology and its application to radiology will be interesting to observe in the next few years. The new technology is apparently making great strides in reducing the amount of radiation to which patients must be exposed. With this development, we can expect to see increased utilization of radiological technology in the diagnostic and treatment processes.

Refinements of ultrasound technology and usage will also present new horizons for the radiologist. There are indications that this method is being groomed as a replacement for today's traditional exploratory surgery. By having a clearer picture of prevailing conditions within the body prior to surgery, the surgeon will be better able to limit his procedure to the precise area of need, reducing the lengths of surgical hospitalization.

Radiologists may also expect additional refinements in the precision of radiation therapy for cancer, making this method more effective and of greater value in the fight against a dreaded killer.

As the field of electronics becomes increasingly sophisticated, reducing the size and price of many units, the availability and versatility of radiology equipment are expected to improve markedly.

What will be the total impact of these changes? Thanks to all of these improvements, the increased use of radiological services would seem to be an inevitable result. Though the improvements in efficiency will be substantial, the rising demand for services will place a considerable dent in the improvement. A busier, more automated radiology department will be the likely byproduct for most hospitals across the country.

The greatest challenge for administrative acumen will come from the problem of funding. Who will pay for these improvements? And, will they be willing to pay the price that is required? This is the only real cloud over the advance of radiological process as we enter the last decades of this century.

The Radiology Department: Some Final Thoughts

As one of the greatest allies to the practicing physician or surgeon, the efficient operation of the radiology department is an indispensable part of today's healing science. Though our emphasis has been, and will continue to be, the improvement of operations, we must not permit ourselves to lose sight of the fundamental purposes which we seek to maintain.

With each new development that is implemented by the radiologist, we must pay a certain price. The most difficult portion of the problem comes in striking a balance between the financial needs of the department and the social responsibility to provide top quality health care to the people who need it.

No one disagrees with the basic humanitarian ethic of health care delivery. Our task, which may become a matter of government mandate in the future, is to be certain that portions of our society are not priced out of the health care market.

In the final analysis, enhancing the efficiency of the radiology department could be considered the largest step toward the humanitarian objective, permitting us to maintain effective cost containment goals. If you can work effectively with your hospital's radiologist, the objective of an optimum efficiency radiology department for your hospital will definitely be an attainable goal. *

---

* See also ¶5601 *et seq.,* Prentice-Hall *Hospital Cost Management Service.*

Organizing an efficient hospital pharmacy 15

AS A MAJOR SOURCE OF ADMINISTRATIVE CONCERN in terms of cost controls, few places in the hospital would rival the pharmacy department. With a spiraling of pharmaceutical costs and regulatory red tape, the challenge presented here can overshadow many other areas of hospital administration.

Because of its high visibility within the hospital's clinical mission, as well as the nature of substances under its jurisdiction, the pharmacy is under the tightest controls of any department within the hospital. As the number of pharmaceutical compounds proliferates, along with increased potencies which can be developed, the concerns of the Legal Community have been centered on the potential dangers of improper pharmacy management.

This legal concern has been elevated to a major area of administrative consideration due to the trend toward incorporating pharmaceutical requirements into the total hospital licensure picture. This interconnection was designed to force closer administrative oversight of hospital pharmaceutical activities.

As these legal considerations become increasingly constraining, the need for direct administrative control virtually compels many hospitals to initiate an in-hospital pharmacy program. As opposed to the "consulting service" pharmacist, the in-house pharmacy offers many advantages from an administrative and cost control viewpoint. These advantages make an in-hospital pharmacy a virtual necessity for all but the smallest hospitals in the country.

During the course of this chapter, we hope to give sufficient details to enable your hospital either to establish a pharmacy or improve the operations of your current setup. The cost savings could be sufficiently dramatic to ease the upward pressures on your daily operating costs.

In-house vs. Consulting Service: A Question of Cost

Establishing a full-service hospital pharmacy is definitely not an inexpensive endeavor. This fact alone has tended to prevent a large number of hospitals from initiating the program, despite some obvious long-term benefits. As mentioned earlier, some of the smallest hospitals may not experience major cost benefits from an in-house pharmacy. But, for all the rest, the benefits definitely outweigh the initial investments required to start the program.

Though definitive guidelines may be somewhat hard to formulate, we might go out on a limb and offer this generalized guideline:

BED CAPACITY	BEST COURSE OF ACTION
50 or less	Probably best to keep consulting service.
50 to 100	This is the marginal area. Either one, depending on hospital's financial picture.
100 or more	In-hospital pharmacy definitely recommended.

From a cost standpoint, the major problem with the consulting service pharmacist system lies in the fact that the hospital must continually deal with a *retail pharmaceuticals merchant*. Though costs may be somewhat less than what the standard "off the street' customer encounters, basically due to the quantities involved, these pharmacists are definitely businessmen first. They aren't in the business for their health. The profits they reap from a hospital's business represent additional costs for your operations.

If this approach is modified, with the hospital purchasing pharmaceuticals from the wholesaler, the consulting service pharmacist is likely to take lost profits into account in determining the amount of his retainer fee for services to your hospital.

With either alternative, the control of the pharmacy's administrative costs is literally out of your hands. Because the consulting service pharmacist will often have an independent pharmacy outside the hospital, he is less subject to administrative direction and control in daily operations. As long as the pharmacist operates within the contraints of state and federal laws, there is little you can do to influence his operations.

If you should decide to attempt to exercise more than an absolute minimum of administrative oversight, and are seen as excessively meddling in the pharmacy business, the pharmacist may shout an unprintable expletive, graphically describe where you can put your pharmacy, and literally leave you "holding the bag" on its daily operations. This type of insecurity is definitely no way to effectively administer hospital operations.

By contrast, an in-hospital pharmacy makes the pharmacist a salaried member of the hospital staff. This fact alone makes him far more susceptible to administrative direction. Without the outside business benefits, financial health becomes a constraining factor in the pharmacist's attitude. Because his job would be on the line, this pharmacist would be likely to observe tighter cost constraints on his department, offering considerable benefits to the hospital.

In addition, the salaried pharmacist is not motivated by a personal profit in daily operations. While this might occasionally represent a negative factor, reducing the pharmacist's initiative, the overall effect is a positive one. Quality control would never be sacrificed for the sake of an extra dollar, which might be the case in the other system.

On balance, the in-hospital pharmacy system is definitely the preferable route. To illustrate this, let's consider the following case history which shows a very dramatic result in establishing an in-hospital pharmacy.

CASE IN POINT: ESTABLISHING HOSPITAL PHARMACY SLASHES OVER 20 PERCENT ON PHARMACEUTICAL COSTS

For one midwestern hospital, the standard method of operations for several decades had been to purchase pharmaceuticals from area pharmacies, accepting the deals which could be made with them. Though this system had been established while the hospital was small, no one had taken the time to review the situation, even though the hospital's size had subsequently more than doubled.

Under new administrative direction, one of the first priorities was to check into all available alternatives for operating the hospital's pharmaceutical activities. After examining the problem, the administration decided to set up their own in-hospital pharmacy.

Thanks to the establishment of excellent ties with wholesale pharmaceutical companies and first-rate pharmacy management, the results after two years of operation were impressive. Counting the salary factor for the pharmacist, the net savings on pharmaceutical services for the hospital were an astonishing 22 percent.

The results of the above case history, while not necessarily a standard result from this move, do show the positive nature of results which can be obtained. While some portion of the savings could be attributed to the fact that pharmaceuticals were previously purchased on the retail market, at least half of the total savings could be attributed to the increased efficiencies which result from having the pharmacy operation originating inside the hospital's walls.

Pharmacy Authority Structure

As an adjunct service to the practice of medicine, the fundamental authority for pharmacy services, by law and by common standards of efficiency, originates from the hospital's medical staff. Under the physicians' direct supervision, the pharmaceutical function is an increasingly valuable ally of the healing sciences.

As a semi-autonomous hospital department, the policy formulations for the pharmacy are instituted through the combined efforts of varied members of the medical staff, the pharmacist in charge, and the hospital's administration. These three areas are commonly represented on the policy-making panel which governs all pharmaceutical activities for the hospital.

The Pharmacy and Therapeutics Committee, as the policy panel is often referred to, meets a minimum of two times annually (and holds such additional meetings as are necessary) to discuss the essential business and policy considerations which involve the operations of the hospital pharmacy. In addition to standard policy, the committee is also responsible for deciding which medications are to be permitted in the hospital, evaluates data on medications currently in use, and serves as a watchdog bureaucracy to avoid duplication of drugs or other similar causes of pharmaceutical cost overruns.

When operated according to the design for such committees, it can serve as a complete advisory agency for the top-flight implementation of pharmaceutical practice within the hospital.

The Pharmacist's Role

For the chief of a hospital's pharmacy, the role of organizer and main monitor of pharmaceutical supplies is the primary responsibility. This organization is the key element to maintaining efficient operations for his department.

In capsulized form to fit our discussion, let's briefly list the standard roles and functions which are the specific domain of the hospital's chief pharmacist.

   (1) The dispensing of all hospital drugs.
   (2) Preparation of all injectable substances, when such manufacture of combination medications is performed in the hospital.
   (3) Filling and labeling of all medication containers for services which dispense them to patients.
   (4) Inspection of all pharmaceuticals housed in all hospital services.
   (5) Maintaining stocks of antidotes and other emergency medications.
   (6) Developing and maintaining specifications for all drugs, chemicals, biologicals, antibiotics, and any other pharmaceutical preparations. (Specifications refer to quality of product and source of supply.)
   (7) Maintaining hospital's narcotics and alcohol control program.
   (8) Furnishing pharmaceutical information to the hospital's medical and nursing staffs.
   (9) The establishment and maintenance of adequate accounting and records procedures for pharmacy charges and supply requisitions.
 (10) Planning and directing pharmacy policy.
 (11) Facilities maintenance.
 (12) In teaching hospitals: cooperation with the nursing and/or medical school in teaching courses involving pharmaceuticals.

(13) Implementing decisions rendered by the Pharmacy and Therapeutics Committee.

(14) Furnishing written reports on pharmacy activities to the hospital's administrator.

The functions listed above also form the essential core of hospital pharmaceutical policy. The most important aspect of the operations, though, is the control of dispensed pharmaceuticals and maintenance of adequate records to enable the pharmacist to account for every bit of medication which leaves the pharmacy. We do not exaggerate in stating that failure to monitor this area effectively could literally put a hospital out of business.

CASE IN POINT: HOSPITAL LICENSE SUSPENDED FOR PHARMACY VIOLATIONS— STATE CLOSES HOSPITAL'S DOORS

In a case which received some exposure in the news media, one western hospital was confronted with a problem involving the control of medications within its confines. As a direct result, some very adverse effects were felt in the clinical care area.

When the administration failed to examine the situation more closely, and after complaints were registered by certain hospital staff members, state officials conducted an investigation of the situation. Finding negligence on the part of both the hospital's pharmacy and its administration, the investigating officials ordered the current patients transferred to other hospitals and the doors of the offending hospital closed.

Though there is some differential in state laws inolving the control of pharmaceuticals, few states, if any, will permit a substantial breakdown in the drug monitoring system. This position is totally justifiable for public safety reasons. Consider the fact that the above case illustration *resulted in numerous patient deaths.*

Because much of the procedural policy for pharmacy operation is dictated by a variety of state and federal regulations, a discussion of precise policy specifics is probably not suitable for our purposes here. The effort to offer policy guidelines might present points which are contrary to a state regulation where your hospital is located.

We can, however, emphasize that efficiency is best served by keeping policy points to an absolute minimum. A simple mechanism will almost always perform more efficiently than a complex one. As permitted by the laws governing your hospital's pharmaceutical activities, make every effort to streamline the department's policies. This could pay off in substantial dividends for the future.

Pharmacy Facilities

Though the overall size of the pharmacy's facilities is most often determined by its total workload, the facilities must be adequate to provide room for the basics of pharmaceutical service. The primary space consumers in most hospital pharmacies involve equipment for compounding, manufacturing, and dispensing prescribed medications and the space needed for standard and refrigerated storage of pharmaceuticals.

Additional space is required to house the necessary administrative paraphernalia; record-keeping supplies, filing equipment, etc.

The final requirement, though definitely not the least important, is that there is adequate floor space to permit uncramped operations. This is particularly important in larger, busier hospital pharmacies involving numerous staff members working in the same room.

Security Problems

One major problem facing hospital pharmacies, particularly those located in high-crime metropolitan areas, involves maintaining security for controlled substances; narcotics, hallucinogens, etc. With the spiral of "street value" for illicitly obtained drugs, hospital pharmacies can become a prime target for theft-minded drug addicts, pushers looking for a source of supply with 100 percent profit, or even influences from the organized crime sector.

Regardless of the source, the problem can become a major source of concern for hospital administrators. Due to their value, the losses of a single theft could prove devastating to a hospital's financial picture.

CASE IN POINT: DRUG THEFT NETS THREE-QUARTER MILLION DOLLARS

Located in a relatively high-crime rate area, one midwestern metropolitan hospital was being hit by a series of small thefts of controlled substances from their pharmacy. Though there was some effort made to determine the identity of the thieves, no major changes were instituted to make the department more secure from this menace. According to the hospital's administrator, the losses were not "sufficiently significant" to warrant drastic action.

This quickly changed when, in a daring night raid on the basement pharmacy facilities, the entire stock of narcotics, worth in excess of $750,000, was stolen.

Shocked by this sudden clean-out of its pharmacy, the hospital's administrator and governing board called in a professional security consultant. After examining the situation, the consultant directed that the pharmacy be relocated on the hospital's first floor, close to regular traffic patterns which are maintained 24 hours a day. In addition, a thick-walled combination safe (equipped with burglar alarm) was built into one wall of the new pharmacy facility. The same setup was also instituted for the refrigeration unit. These three improvements were designed to reduce the accessibility of the hospital's pharmaceutical inventory.

As a direct result of these changes, the ongoing pattern of pharmaceutical thefts was halted completely. After the new pharmacy facility was completed and put into operation, not a single bit of controlled substances has been stolen from the hospital. This phenominal record has been maintained for over THREE YEARS.

This case history clearly illustrates the basic fundamentals involved in maintaining a hospital pharmacy's security in the face of outside threats. To re-cap the highlights of the case history, the following points contribute to increased security:

(1) Centralized location within normally heavy traffic corridors.
(2) Adequate alarm systems to serve as a deterrent.
(3) Modifying the standard mode of equipment installation (the wall inset idea) to make theft of pharmaceuticals more difficult.
(4) Storage facility walls sufficiently thick to be virtually impenetrable to forced entry.

If these four points are judiciously implemented in your pharmacy, the potential for security problems should be markedly less. Though the initial investment may seem high to implement improvements, the results of one successful robbery could easily wipe out any positive financial benefits of failing to bolster security.

Additional Pharmacy Staffing

In addition to the chief pharmacist, your hospital's workload may require added staff for the department. Depending on the regulations for your state, these may be either assistants or added registered pharmacists. In either case, the ratio of one pharmacy staff member for each 50 beds of hospital capacity is a fairly accurate staffing estimate. Though this may vary somewhat, the general consensus is that a ratio of more patients per pharmacist could ultimately prove detrimental to long-term departmental efficiency objectives.

For smaller hospitals, particularly those under 100 beds, the problem of adequate pharmacy staff utilization can prove to be a stumbling block. While the need for an in-house pharmacy is evident, the problem of slack periods can prove vexing.

Two potential solutions which appear to offer hope involve; (1) assigning other duties as, for instance, in the lab, or (2) having two nearby hospitals sharing the services of one pharmacist, working for each on a part-time basis.

The Battle over "Generics"

If one wished to witness a vociferous argument, all that would be required is to mention "generic" drugs to a group of physicians. This subject has been the center of a heated controversy between consumer groups, the medical profession, and pharmaceutical manufacturers.

Essentially, the major difference between the so-called "generic" medication and any others is the lack of a brand name on the product. Because the standards and regulations imposed on the manufacture of all pharmaceuticals within the United

States are so stringent, a large percentage of pharmacists agree that there is little, if any, difference between generic and regular drugs as it pertains to quality.

From an administrative standpoint, the generic pharmaceuticals can offer substantial advantages in terms of cost. The lack of advertising on these generic drugs has a positive, lowering effect on prices. When the major pharmaceutical companies advertise their new drugs (and ongoing products) in the medical journals, along with their company representatives passing out their "free" samples, someone has to pick up the tab for these promotional costs.

The end result is that the hospital and, ultimately, the patient must bear the burden for these promotional costs, all incorporated into the final price for the product.

If, as the pharmacists seem to agree, there is so little difference between the two drug classifications, why is there so much resistance to the generic idea? Some of the problem could probably be traced to a form of psychological identification with certain brand names.

As an example, consider the *generic term* "Facial Tissues." How many of us will ask for the facial tissue? Instead, isn't it more likely that we'll say, "Could you bring me a KLEENEX?" The word has become synonymous for the words, facial tissue.

This same form of identification has been impressed on the medical community by skillful pharmaceutical house salesmen. Particularly true of the larger, more established companies, they have successfully substituted their brand names for the regular product names as the symbol of quality. This statement is not intended as defamatory of the major drug manufacturers. It is merely a statement of reality.

How can you, as administrator, ever hope to circumvent this problem? Initially, you must recognize the source of the problem for what it really is, a psychological identification process. Using the gentle art of persuasion, with statistics to back up your claims, attempt to make a gradual transition from the name-brand market to the generics. Possibly trying out on one or two medications, you can gradually begin to "wean" the medical staff from the brands they identify with.

As long as the incoming generics meet the standards and specifications which your hospital requires for its pharmaceuticals, there should be no sacrifice in the quality of care that patients receive.

The matter of cost can be substantially different, however. Even in smaller lots, as sold to consumers, the generic pharmaceuticals can offer 20 percent to 30 percent reductions as opposed to the standard brand names. In the larger quantities which hospitals often purchase, the savings can be even more dramatic.

The only real challenge lies in maintaining an intricate psychological balance during the transition process. This balance is extremely important in avoiding unnecessary antagonisms which can prove disruptive to other procedures and to general hospital staff morale.

If this can be avoided, the positive impact of this change could serve as the centerpiece of efforts to implement effective cost containment practices for health care delivery in your hospital.

Paper Work Requirements

As in every other hospital department, there are some basic record-keeping paper work items for the pharmacy which can never be overlooked. Though much of this workload is dictated by laws and regulations, our continuing emphasis on simplification of processes is not being overlooked.

The basic essentials for the pharmacy can be encompassed in a relatively few selected forms. Written inventory listings for all pharmaceuticals, a definite requirement by law, can be accomplished with a fairly simple form. This would have a listing of the most commonly used hospital drugs preprinted on the form with space provided for entering quantities.

The form would also have space to list the less commonly used drugs, with a pharmacy staff member writing in the drug names in blank spaces provided. By preprinting the most common ones, the amount of writing required is substantially reduced.

This type of inventory form should be a "special design" model to conform to the individual requirements of your hospital, not a standard design form which might be available from a printing company or pharmaceutical company. These standard forms are not tailor-made to your needs and do not enhance the efficiency of your pharmacy's operations.

As the supply of inventory forms is depleted, you might find it advisable to convene a meeting of your pharmacy and therapeutics committee to review the inventory form's contents. If new medications are used to replace old standards, this fact should be reflected on the inventory form. A degree of administrative flexibility can go a long way toward enhancing pharmacy operations here.

In addition to inventory forms, special narcotics order forms purchased from the Internal Revenue Service, standard pharmaceutical order forms, internal stock requisition and control forms, and reports for administrative use round out the picture.

The most important of the administrative reports is the annual recounting of pharmacy activities for the Administrator's inspection. This annual report has three general parts; (1) Financial status, (2) Re-cap of activities and accomplishments, and (3) Plans for any changes and/or improvements in the coming year.

Under the second category, specific information on quantities of prescriptions and nursing unit baskets filled must be provided. In addition, the report must contain information on the in-house manufacturing program, educational programs, activities of the pharmacy and therapeutics committee, changes in the hospital's drug lists, and results of any unit inspections conducted by the pharmacy during the previous year.

This report serves to underscore the value of the hospital's pharmacy to the overall objectives of administrative policy. It is often used as the basis for policy decisions which directly affect pharmacy operations, including approved allotments for the department in the total hospital budget.

Final Thoughts on the Pharmacy

Hospital pharmacy operations are, by necessity, fairly complex entities. The high visibility in the clinical picture, as mentioned at the beginning of this chapter, makes efficiency a top priority for this department. Any breakdown here will have an adverse effect on the public's confidence in your hospital.

Most important, we wish to emphasize the idea of simplifying the operations to the greatest degree possible. Any excessive administrative "wrinkles" which are incorporated into the system will only serve to deter the efficiency objective.

The real key to a pharmacy's success is the dedication of its staff to the objectives of clinical excellence and administrative plan implementation. The pharmacy, despite its apparent autonomy, must not lose sight of its role as team player in hospital planning.

If a spirit of cooperation and essential communication are maintained between the pharmacy and other departments which need its services, the efficiencies made possible by an in-hospital pharmacy will prove to be a major contributor to the building and continuation of your hospital's success. *

---

* See also ¶8401 *et seq.,* Prentice-Hall *Hospital Cost Management Service.*

Dynamic management concepts for dietary services 16

FOOD, THE BASIC STAPLE OF DAILY LIVING outside of the hospital, plays an integral role in a multi-faceted, scientifically based health improvement program for the patients housed at your hospital. The dietary service serves this role through a dual approach which serves the physical maintenance and health-building aspects of the food preparation regimen.

The two-part design of dietary service demands that a dual-authority structure is established to effectively handle the two basic functions of the department. The two authority positions involved are the Dietician and the Food Service Manager.

From a scientific viewpoint, the dietician plays the more dominant role in the dietary service planning prospectus. The dietician, through training and experience, has the background to formulate the hospital's menu to meet specific medical and scientific objectives. This one factor serves as the major distinction between the positions of dietician and food service manager.

By contrast, the food service manager is the *implementer* of dietary service management planning, helping to monitor the incidental details of the service's daily operations. Working from the established monthly and annual budgets for the service, the food service manager's objective is to keep operations at an acceptable per capita cost level based on the Hospital Census. The challenge is to accomplish this while, at the same time, serving food which is acceptable to patients' palates.

While the dietician is termed the head of this department (for organizational purposes), it is the effective operation of the dual-authority structure which assures the best interests of the dietary service. The efficient coordination of the combined medical and administrative concerns in operating this department will assure that its maximum potential contribution to the total hospital health care scenario can be fully realized.

This chapter, in addition to examining the specific roles of the dietician and the food service manager, pinpoints the daily operational problems most apt to create the greatest difficulties. You will be offered some hospital-tested potential solutions—some to be considered rather innovative—which could effectively reduce the common problems of dietary department operations.

The Dietician's Role

In some smaller hospital operations, the positions of dietician and food service manager are combined into one position under the dietician title. Payoff: This combined position will have the duties described in this subsection *plus* those which appear in the portion devoted to the food service manager. At this point, we will focus on the role of the dietician as a single position.

The single-role dietician performs her duties from a scientific basis to correlate the hospital's food preparation and serving with the medical objectives which are sought by the hospital's physicians. With a background of specialized training in nutrition, her function becomes the selection of foods which will be of the greatest benefit to the patient. This is of particular value to those patients with specialized dietary needs; i.e., diabetes, ulcers, etc.

In most hospitals, physicians delegate the responsibility of explaining the importance of, and the technical aspects concerning, the diets which patients must follow when they leave the hospital. If the dietician's background is sufficient, the doctor may decide to permit her to design the patients' diets based on available information on pertinent medical conditions and with minimal professional supervision.

As a practical matter pertaining to daily departmental operations, the dietician must be the "Chief of Staff" for the food preparation process. The dietician's rule must be supreme to assure that patients receive the appropriate allotments and variety in the foods which are served.

For administrative purposes, put the dietician in direct communication with the business office to assure that accurate information regarding patient numbers is maintained by the dietary department. This information prevents the possibility of inadvertent food shortages due to inadequate amounts being prepared. By the same token, this also reduces the potential for waste by controlling the amounts based on the Patient Census.

From the medical information viewpoint, maintain contact with the nursing service, the medical staff, and the medical records areas. This keeps the food selection process on a scientific basis, working from the most current information on patients and their progress in treatment. These variables, while most important to the medical aspect, also play a large role in the administrative aspect of departmental operation. Changes in diagnosis could result in some significant changes in dietary methods for a patient.

In addition to the theoretical applications of established dietary practice, the dietician should take an active role in the food procurement process, regardless of whether or not a food service manager has been retained for the department. By keeping informed of the food picture, particularly as it applies to seasonal availability, the dietician can be more effective in hospital menu-planning for general and special diets.

Because the availability of competently trained dieticians does not appear to be keeping pace with the demand for their services, a hospital may be required to settle for a part-time or consulting-service dietician to serve the hospital. This idea, particularly if it is through an established shared-service agreement with another hospital, still provides adequate service for the patients. The shared-service plan also offers substantial benefits in the cost containment area, a major concern for smaller hospital dietary services.

In such cases, the food service manager becomes the de facto head of the dietary service, performing all other duties except those directly related to the medical decision-making realm. This area would be reserved for the dietician or, in extreme cases, for more direct participation by members of the hospital's medical staff.

If no trained dietician is available for the hospital, the problem might be circumvented by the appointment of one medical staff member as part-time monitor and general consultant for the dietary service. This is not the ideal solution for two basic reasons.

First, there is likely to be a considerable amount of resistance from physicians to having additional duties heaped on them. In most hospitals, they have sufficient duties available to keep them more than adequately occupied.

Second, there is a general consensus by trained hospital observers that most physicians do not have sufficient background in dietary sciences to fully serve the best interests of their patients. This statement is not meant as a deprecation of the medical profession, but merely a recognition of the specialized nature of dietary planning.

Nutrition, particularly as it applies to the healing sciences, is an exacting realm. Most medical schools do not provide extensive training in dietary sciences because it's assumed that a dietician will be available to handle the food selection and planning process. This, unfortunately, is not always the order of the day.

For our purposes, our objective should be to retain, at least on a part-time basis, the services of a competent professional dietician to meet patients' needs. The second important requirement is administrative ability. Because food preparation and its service to patients could represent a substantial percentage of a hospital's expenses, if not managed properly, effective administration of the dietary service is a vital link in maintaining a positive posture for the hospital's final balance sheet.

To this end, the dietician must be responsible for proper completion of department records which are turned in to the business office. These records would include periodic accounting of department activities, requisitions for required foods, and, in the cases of auxiliary dietary services performed by the hospital's department, an accurate accounting of meals served to facilitate proper weekly or monthly billing practices.

As a final item, the dietician should be responsible for (though it is potentially delegated within the department) the inventory practice to assure adequate supplies and records of supply usage. The averages compiled through this method will give the dietician a fairly accurate picture of departmental operations to facilitate the preparation of the dietary service's annual budget.

In essence, the administrative and scientific details of the dietary service's function are the specific domain of the hospital's dietician. For all practical purposes, this is the *only* way that appropriate quality can be assured.

The Food Service Manager

In contrast to the dietician, the food service manager deals with the technical aspects of the daily food delivery system. Translating the orders of the dietician and the attending physicians into concrete action is a vital consideration in the efficiency picture.

As a middle management position (except in the absence of a professional dietician), food service management must deal with the details which, though often unseen, are only noteworthy in their absence. Some examples would include food storage procedures, kitchen equipment maintenance, appropriate sanitation procedures for facilities and utensils, monitoring the performance of staff members, and the delegation of duties for auxiliary dietary department functions—such as the proper maintenance of hospital vending machines.

The background of the food service manager should definitely include solid training in the area of home economics, preferably through college-based training. While the college-educated food service manager would definitely require more pay than a person with a lesser background, the additional benefits derived from the enhanced education will pay substantial dividends to the employing hospital.

Aside from the technical aspects of dealing with dietary service equipment, the greatest area of challenge for the food service manager comes from the supervisory role which the job requires. Facing similar problems as other departmental supervisors, food service managers must be a combination of amateur psychologist and "slave driver" in an attempt to gain maximum productivity from the employees under her command.

The manager's analytical ability should be able to decipher whether lagging productivity is due to some problem with the employees or a lack of appropriate equipment to get the job done. In either case, the food service manager's obligation is to assure the correction of the problem or problems involved.

Staffing Levels

A slight twist on an old saying, "All Chiefs and no Indians makes for a chaotic tribe," applies to the structure of the hospital's dietary service. Despite some notable advances in equipment technology, supervisory personnel alone could never provide adequate levels of service to any hospital when it comes to food service.

Most knowledgeable observers place the staffing level for dietary services at one staffer per five beds of hospital capacity. While all of these people would not be in the kitchen itself, a good portion would be involved directly in the food preparation process. One major reason that staffing levels are so high stems from the *low* pay which is commonly assigned to dietary help. With low pay, the quality of available help tends to be rather low, favoring the transient type of individual. Residual problems from a high turnover rate contribute to reduced efficiency and major increases in expenses.

By a reverse sort of logic, the dietary service can actually be operated on *less* money if its employees are paid *more*. While this may, on the surface, seem to be contradictory, there are several solid reasons why this situation would actually work in the hospital's favor.

In order to promote departmental efficiency, our objective should be to keep employees around long enough to learn their jobs thoroughly and to help your hospital to gain the benefits of this knowledge. The higher pay would achieve this objective.

A second point is the matter of "professional" image. If an employee can associate his or her job with a type of professionalism, a greater amount of job satisfaction can be expected. People who are satisfied with their jobs are less likely to wish for other employment. Higher pay levels contribute to this objective.

The third, and final, point is probably the most important. When your hospital's dietary service acquires a reputation for paying better wages, the quality of available applicants is certain to rise. Your dietician or food service manager will not be forced to settle for marginal abilities in potential employees. This helps to speed up the transition process of new employees to the jobs involved, effectively reducing the extent of inefficiencies which inevitably result from employee transition periods.

The only remaining question becomes, "Does this theory work in actual practical application?" The answer is an unqualified "Yes." Here's one case study which serves to illustrate the idea in action.

CASE IN POINT: WAGE INCREASE PLAN WORKS "MAGIC" IN STREAMLINING MIDWESTERN METROPOLITAN HOSPITAL'S DIETARY SERVICE.

Afflicted with employee transiency and a higher than expected staffing level to provide needed food services, one midwestern hospital decided to take the radical step of increasing wages for the service by 15 percent. One objective of the plan, according to the administrator, was to see if a higher pay scale might encourage better productivity from the current staff members.

Another reason for the move, well-publicized in the local media, was to attract a broader range of applicants for positions which were being advertised for the dietary service. The plan began to pay off immediately.

The first dividend came from employee attitude. When some job titles were altered, along with the better pay, to give the tasks a more professional appearance, dietary service staff members began to take a more constructive interest in the department's function. The better-quality intellects in the group became more inspired to make suggestions and to *prove* their professionalism on the job. In a process quite similar to separating the chaff from the wheat, the less dependable transients continued to depart as before, leaving the quality employees behind.

The second payoff came in the quality of the new applicants. They, like the employees who remained, were of better quality. Stable citizens from within the hospital's own community began applying for jobs with the dietary service. It was no longer considered to be a second-class job, to be accepted when nothing else was available.

Within 18 months, the complete transition to a quality staff revealed that staff numbers could be reduced by over 20 percent. From a level of 1 staffer for every 4 beds of capacity, this was reduced to 1 staffer per 5.2 beds of capacity.

Though this meant that 29 fewer employees were involved for this 510-bed facility, there was no reduction in the quality of dietary services. In fact, by some internal estimations, the addition of a 40-bed, extended-care facility to the hospital complex could be accomplished *with no additional dietary staff help required.*

The facts from this case study speak for themselves. The perennial consumers' axiom, "You get what you pay for," is nowhere more true than in the quality of your dietary staff. Reversing the traditional rule of thumb regarding dietary staff wages could pay equally large dividends for your hospital as well.

Contracted Services for Dietary

Contracted services for a hospital's dietary department are a subject that most administrators, at some point, are prone to consider. If the contract offered by the service provider is attractive, this can be a major temptation. The idea of bypassing potential labor troubles through this route can draw even the most adamant opponent of contract service plans into considering the option. For the small hospital, the idea could be considered as a positive move due to the investment which dietary service equipment would require. This one factor makes the plan of solid merit for the 50-bed to 100-bed hospital.

The major source of problems with this arrangement comes from maintaining this program for a prolonged period. While the cash outlay for maintaining the program departs in a piecemeal fashion, the long-term impact on the hospital's expense picture can be quite negative. Over a period of 10 to 15 years, the program could prove to be much more expensive than if a dietary service had been established in the first place.

Contract services for the dietary department could be, at best, considered as a transitional device. By delaying the overall investment for dietary equipment until a hospital is on more solid ground financially, the program can prevent overburdening a hospital's debt picture. When financing for a dietary department can be accomplished in the most advantageous fashion for the hospital, the contracted dietary service should be discontinued in favor of the in-house departmental program. This transition is the surest way to assure the positive impact of establishing a hospital dietary program.

Centralized vs. Decentralized: A Question of Staffing

The relative merits of the centralized dietary service and the decentralized mode have been argued by management theorists as long as hospitals have been providing one of the two alternatives to their patients. Depending on the management expert one consults, either system offers substantial advantages over the other.

In terms of use popularity, the centralized system for distributing food to patients appears to have a substantial lead. The one basic advantage of the centralized system is that it maintains the dietary department's autonomy in hospital operations. Since staff is not drawn from regular floor crews, there is no noticeable reduction in efficiency for regular care operations.

This factor also represents a "flip side" of the financial "coin." Because a minimum number of staffers are required to dispense food to patients, this means that more staffing is needed for the dietary service under the centralized system than in using the decentralized mode.

The decentralized system brings the food on carts to the floors where it's to be served, in bulk, with the dispensing and service being accomplished by the floor aides and members of the nursing staff. By detracting from these staff members' regular duties, there is a distinct possibility that other equally important functions could be sacrificed—or force an increase in staffing for the floor aide sector.

When all factors are considered, the centralized system, with food coming to individual floors ready to be dispensed to patients, offers the greatest advantages with the least potential disruption to regular floor staff functions. In our opinion, this is probably the method of greatest merit for most currently developed hospital designs in use today.

Feeding the Hired Help

The successful feeding of a hospital's patients usually does not mean the end of the dietary service's obligation. The employees of the hospital, including the medical staff, are usually provided meals by the dietary service. As a matter of tradition, this has been policy for most hospitals covering a period of several decades.

This tradition has represented a major problem for dietary service planning. As the costs of providing essential services escalate, innovative planning ideas become a necessity to provide adequate dietary service at costs which remain at reasonable levels.

One new idea has been to increase the reliance on self-service methods for dispensing food to employees. Though, on the surface, this appears to place a premium on employee honesty, a proper monitoring system removes the risk factor while slashing the number of dietary service employees involved in dispensing food to fellow hospital staffers.

To underscore the importance of this innovation in management planning, let's take a look at one case in which this idea was implemented, along with the results which the program obtained.

**CASE IN POINT: STREAMLINED EMPLOYEE CAFETERIA SYSTEM
SLASHES 10 PERCENT FROM EASTERN HOSPITAL'S
DIETARY SERVICE COSTS.**

With the demands of hospital patient service increasing, along with the attendant price tag, one eastern hospital decided to revamp its cafeteria system to reduce demands on dietary service staff. Under the old system, a considerable reliance was placed on dietary staff serving meals to hospital employees. This method tied up valuable people who could have been utilized more productively in other departmental functions.

The revamped service placed a far greater emphasis on the self-service angle, incorporating a full salad bar for employee use and reducing the variety of hot dishes available for an individual meal. This was followed by the use of vending machines for some food items which could be practically adapted to this system. The idea was to make hospital employees more responsible for serving their own meals, to the extent that such an arrangement could be implemented. After some changes in procedure, dietary staff participation in employee meals was limited to two people, including the cashier who handled the meal cards or cash payments (depending on the employee's preference in the matter).

The end result of the program was a major improvement of dietary services to all segments of the hospital's population at a savings of over $40,000 a year. This figure represented approximately 10 percent of the dietary service's annual budget.

The system's changes were mainly a matter of floor plan arrangement, with only an investment of slightly over $1,000 required to implement the new employee cafeteria program.

This case study makes a strong argument for departing from traditional methods of operation in favor of new ideas which can help to slash overhead expenses. This particular method was an exceptional success because of two factors not mentioned in the case history. The first factor is the ready acceptance of the new system by the hospital staff. A major amount of staff resistance to the new format could have effectively sabotaged the entire plan.

The second factor is the conscientiousness of the few dietary staff members assigned to employee food service. If the staff members had not increased their monitoring vigilance under the self-service plan, the distinct possibility of unaccounted-for employee meals could have happened.

While the implementation of this idea could present some potential difficulties, efforts of this nature or of similar structure which are designed to streamline procedures and reduce operating costs should definitely be encouraged. The main criterion is to be certain that the results retain an equivalent, or bring an enhanced, quality service for your hospital.

Supplementary Revenue-Producing Programs

In an overall hospital drive to acquire additional revenue, the dietary service is admirably equipped to make a substantial contribution to management objectives.

If, as a result of departmental analysis, there are solid indications that some spare time exists which could be productively utilized, the high-quality dietary service can offer an extremely marketable product to surrounding facilities. Some potential ideas in this area might include preparing meals for schools, elders' homes, children's day care centers, and even jails. While much of this auxiliary revenue production depends on the level of activity demanded by inpatient services and the efficiency of the dietary service, the capable department has many avenues which a creative administrator and dietician (or food service manager) can capitalize on.

The main benefit of these supplementary revenue production ideas is to enable the financing of expansion without placing an undue burden on the cost structure which must be passed on to a hospital's patients. Due to an increasing vigilance by insurance "watchdog" groups, a hospital's management flexibility could be seriously damaged without these outside revenue producers.

To highlight the potential benefits of innovative marketing strategies for the dietary service, let's take a look at one small program implemented by a midwestern hospital that began providing meals to a nearby jail facility. This one small program was just the beginning of a long-term revenue-producing program for the hospital.

CASE IN POINT: JAIL INMATE FEEDING PROGRAM GROSSES OVER $11,000 ANNUALLY FOR MIDWESTERN HOSPITAL'S DIETARY SERVICE.

In an effort to generate additional revenue for the facility, one midwestern hospital's dietary service began exploring the marketing of its product to other facilities in their community.

The hospital's dietary service proved to be the perfect solution to a nagging problem plaguing a nearby jail facility which was being pressured to update its meal preparation operations. Due to its small size, averaging only 20 meals per day, the major facility investment for the jail would have been prohibitive.

Exploring this alternative, the law enforcement officials found that they could provide good meals for jailed inmates at slightly over $1.50 per meal. This amounted to less than $11,100 annually. That amount would not have covered the services of a cook, much less take into account the investment for new and improved kitchen equipment.

The deal was made for the hospital to provide meals for the jail. Because the additional revenue helped to modernize the hospital's kitchen, no additional employees were required. No added costs from the modernization had to be passed on to the hospital's patients. Further, the modernization resulted in substantially increased efficiency for other daily operations.

The jail welcomed this arrangement as well. The hospital-provided meal program effectively cut their cost of food preparation and dietary operation by approximately 50 percent, permitting them to meet the new standards without any additional investment for equipment and with the elimination of all in-jail dietary personnel.

This dramatic example of community cooperation between the hospital and other facilities in the area shows that substantial benefits can be realized by the creative food service manager or dietician. By refusing to block the extent of available horizons with limited thinking, this jail dietary program opened the doors to new vistas in innovation for this hospital's dietary service.

Expanded marketing programs permit the dietary service to expand the demand for its services to meet increases in capacity which internal improvements can create. Rather than discharge employees because of efficiency, the emphasis is to get more work to be done.

Frozen Foods: An Analysis

In an effort to improve efficiency, many hospitals are turning to the idea of prepackaged frozen foods to try streamlining the food preparation process. While this can prove to be beneficial from the productivity angle, some negative considerations must be taken into account before major shifts to this food source are made by any hospital's dietary service.

The greatest sngle negative factor appears to be the cost. Whenever a portion of the work is done by a commercial supplier, there is a "value added" markup which automatically affects the cost of the item. The convenience of frozen, prepackaged foods always has an added cost.

This negative factor can be neutralized somewhat through the use of shrewd purchasing practices. In a partial transition to this source, the dietician can concentrate the department's purchases in the autumn season, making larger purchases of commodities which have experienced larger than expected yields during the growing season. More often than not, prices for these items will be considerably lower during the early parts of the selling season than they would be later on in the year. The same principle can be used with meats when climatic conditions or other factors force growers to sell out substantial amounts of their stock. The sudden glutting of the market can dramatically depress prices which must be paid. Purchasing at this time, provided that expected shelf life and the hospital's freezer facilities permit it, can save the dietary budget from the disastrous upward price spiral which inevitably follows the conclusion of a major "sell" order from the growers.

Frozen foods can represent an excellent source of management flexibility for the dietician or the food service manager. If the purchases can be made to conform to long-range dietary planning for the hospital, the savings can, in some cases, exceed 25 percent. The best asset in the utilization of frozen food is a well-informed food service buyer. By taking maximum advantage of market conditions, frozen foods can represent a financial bonanza for the hospital's dietary service.

By the same token, routine purchasing of frozen foods—regardless of market conditions—is definitely NOT recommended. While these purchases may provide culinary variety with traditionally out-of-season food availability, the cost factors could represent a major increase in the dietary service's budget.

Closing Thoughts on Food Service Management

Though a hospital's dietary service may represent only a small fraction of most general operating budgets, the impact of an efficiently operating department can never be minimized. The effect on patients and hospital staff members alike of good food, served courteously and on time, can have major psychological and physiological benefits.

As a contributor to general hospital efficiency, the dietary service's performance can help keep things running smoothly or, in some extreme circumstances, hopelessly snarl other operations while the dietary service attempts to get its act together. The real key to dietary service success is the inspired and dedicated performance of its staff members to standards of professional excellence.

From an administrative viewpoint, the emphasis should be on inspiring productivity—as a matter of pride—from dietary service staffers. With effective leadership from the hospital's administrator and from the department's supervisory positions, the best possible performance for the service can be attained. The objective is to make the department's activities blend efficiently with other hospital functions. If this is achieved, your administrative goal of a positive, efficiency-enhancing dietary service will have been attained. *

---

* See also ¶7101 *et seq.,* Prentice-Hall *Hospital Cost Management Service.*

The two phases of responsible social services planning

17

THE HOSPITAL'S SOCIAL SERVICES DEPARTMENT, unlike most of the other functions performed within the facility, presents a major problem for administrative analysis and judgment regarding its effectiveness to the total health care mission. Because most of the department's activities deal with the intangible aspects of the patient's transition between hospital and home or an extended-care nursing environment, the standard measures of success commonly applied to other hospital departments are not applicable to the area of social services.

To maintain its effectiveness as a transitional mechanism with the hospital's operational plan, the social services department should be operated within two distinct frameworks which encompass its total goal. The primary framework should deal effectively and sympathetically with the problems of the patients and their immediate families as the recovery process evolves. Maintaining a small measure of flexibility can show a sympathetic attitude toward the problems that a patient's family faces, particularly when they must make some major difficult decisions regarding the future care of their relative. By the same token, this flexibility can't be permitted to become so great as to sacrifice hospital standards and cause unacceptable financial risks to the facility. Striking this balance correctly is the major challenge which most hospital social services departments face today.

The second phase of social service function deals with its relation to outside agencies, particularly its connection to government social service agencies. This role becomes particularly critical in cases of child or spouse abuse. Injury cases which show clear indications of sociological basis require community action to help prevent needless suffering and, in some extreme cases, death. Addressing these severe social problems within the community discreetly, in a situation that is quite frequently emotionally volatile, represents the second major challenge to a hospital's social service.

200

To meet the two-phase challenge before it, the hospital social services department should meet certain standards of organization and operation to assure that departmental activities will meet their designated goals. This chapter will pinpoint the factors which contribute to effective departmental operations. We will also devote space for a discussion of the connection between hospital social service and outside social service agencies, putting the emphasis on the portion that directly contribute to success or failure of these vital functions.

As a related item, we will also include details on one of the newest trends in hospital social service planning, the "Intensive Care Program for Relatives" which addresses the special needs presented by the critically ill and dying patients. The program, as one of its peripheral benefits, has expanded the success of organ donor programs for participating facilities.

Organizing Social Services

Unlike any other departmental service within the hospital, the social services department tends to defy the common concepts normally applied to organization for other departments. The infinite variables which are presented by fluctuations in hospital population and the nature of their needs can make a social service department alternately too large or too small.

The extent of social services involvement, as dictated by existing or amended hospital policy, will largely determine the size and organization of the service. Also to be considered are the age demographics of the typical hospital population and the conditions which forced them to seek hospital care. As an example, older patients are more likely to have conditions which require extended care or other rehabilitative services that require a connection with social services. (A more detailed discussion of this role is offered in Chapter 18.)

For this reason, traditional staffing ratios which are used to determine levels for other departments do not apply effectively in this case. One reasonable "yardstick" is to state that a hospital exceeding the 100-bed capacity level should not consider social services department operations with only one trained social worker. Though a one staffer per 100-bed capacity ratio may be an oversimplification of the situation, it does serve as a preliminary point from which to determine feasible alterations as the nature of the hospital population dictates.

In the multi-staffed social services department, one staffer could be selected as the Chief of Social Services (or another applicable title). The direct responsibilities of the chief of social services include supervision of the department's activities and serving as the liaison between Social Services' activities and those of other hospital departments. This is a vital area of concern because effective hospital management depends greatly on excellent patient transitions from one mode of care to another. This transition enables the hospital to move patients (as medical conditions permit) and open space for new patients as they come in.

In the regulated atmosphere (some might argue that it's over-regulated) of hospital management, the direct connection between the chief of social services and the hospital's Utilization Committee is a most important one. Quite often, the utilization committee effectively sets the priority of action for Social Services as to which patients' cases must be given first attention.

By attempting to balance the physical and psychological needs of a patient with those of the hospital's management objectives, the chief of social services is often "walking a tightrope" between the rival interests. As the public relations "front" for the hospital, the social services department quite often comes in for the "heat" if a patient's transition proves to be a bit premature, possibly causing detrimental effects to the patient's health. Coping with the pressures exerted by the utilization committee—without passing excessive amounts of it on to relatives responsible for the vital decision-making process—can be quite a difficult assignment, even for the most dedicated and level-headed social service worker.

For this reason, selecting the chief of social services involves not only the length of experience in social work. Personal temperament and the ability to deal with pressure effectively should also be prime considerations in the selection process. If the chief of social services is unable to meet the second vital criterion, substantial damage to a hospital's public image and standing in the community is a possibility.

Beyond the role of the chief of social services, make every attempt to have competently trained social workers as subordinate staff members, with the exception of any clerical workers assigned to handle the department's paperwork load. Result: employees who can establish empathy with the people they serve on a daily basis while, at the same time, maintaining a vigilant eye on the management objectives which the hospital wishes to maintain.

The Social Services-Medical Staff Connection

To meet the objectives of hospital utilization, the social services department, by necessity, should maintain an active liaison with the medical staff. This could potentially include the attendance of a department representative at medical staff meetings, along with more direct participation in the functions of the utilization committee. Because the problems of the department are unique, consideration of other facets of the health care delivery team should be given to avoid complicating the department's situation further.

Maintaining an active dialogue between Social Services and other departments through staff meetings and other less formal means is the best way to ease any potential management problems which the department might face. Because the medical staff's decisions regarding patient status have a direct bearing on departmental functions, the dialogue with the medical staff is particularly crucial.

As the centralized "clearinghouse" for information on available alternative care facilities, the social services department is obligated to keep physicians informed as to openings in nursing homes, rehabilitation centers or other similar facilities to enable the medical staff to make intelligent decisions regarding the future statuses of their patients.

Due to their more immediate connection to the psychological well-being of the patients involved, the department must occasionally take exception to some moves recommended by the medical staff, particularly if it involves the transition of a handicapped person from the hospital to the home environment. Because there are often other considerations than the purely medical or managerial objective, these other factors should be pinpointed by the social services department in its communications with the physicians.

As an example, the availability of home care equipment may stall the patient transfer process. No amount of management objective should force a family to take a handicapped and recuperating patient home from the hospital without necessary equipment to permit adequate home care. This could cause adverse results for the physical and psychological health of both the patient and his or her family.

Assisting in this process is usually the role that comes under the duties of the social services department. Thanks to their ongoing connection with suppliers and organizations which can provide special equipment for the handicapped, they are probably in a better position than family members to acquire the needed help quickly and efficiently, sometimes without any direct cost to the patient or the relatives.

Through an effective, ongoing communications process with the medical staff, the social services department may often be able to begin planning for this transition process in advance, enabling an on-schedule transfer of the patient without contributing further to the problems of either the patient or the family. This factor is the primary reason that we must strongly advocate the strengthening of social services-medical staff communications, particularly where it is currently considered a "weak link" in the health care delivery process.

Connections with the Outside

Aside from the necessary arrangements which the social services department would make to assist a patient in the transition process, the hospital's social services department also faces major concerns in other areas which involve outside agencies, either in the social services or law enforcement sector. The most frequent need for this type of connection is in relation to the problems generated by the triad of child abuse, spouse abuse and the crime of rape.

In all of these three, the central issue is the combination of physical and psychological suffering which is inflicted upon the patient. Quite often, the psychological injuries are of the longer duration and may require extensive counseling and help to overcome.

To best serve the patient's interests, the hospital social services department should look to form alliances with counseling groups (either under private sponsorship or government funded) which can help the patient to cope with the mental scarring that often accompanies these acts of violence. Another area of possible liaison is with the so-called "Battered Wives' Shelters" which serve as a protective haven for women who are subjected to a habitual pattern of physical abuse in their homes. Because the problems of spouse abuse and child abuse are so often interrelated, these same shelters offer protection to the children of the unfortunate battered wives.

These special shelters for victims of spouse abuse can represent a major financial help to the hospital, particularly if an effective connection is made between the shelter, county or state social services people, and the hospital's social services department. In many of these cases, the need for immediate physical care passes relatively quickly. But, considering the circumstances surrounding most spouse abuse incidents—and their extreme likelihood to be repeated—which could ultimately have fatal consequences, the hospital could be considered to have abdicated its responsibility to the patient by release to the abuser's custody.

If the prolonged psychological care and sheltered safety are provided by the hospital, this is often done at a major financial loss to the institution. Because abused spouses, most often women, are forced to seek public assistance for an interim period when they first break away from their undesirable situations, the financial reimbursement to the hospital is often dependent on the funds and rules of the government agency.

Due to the limited funding which is often available through these agencies, the financial losses incurred in providing long-term care at reduced rates, frequently applied to care which could be provided elsewhere, can prove staggering. Though the reduced funding proves so adverse to the hospital, the special shelters can operate quite nicely on the agencies' allocations due to their considerably smaller level of overhead. The referral process between hospital and special shelter proves to be a financial bonanza for both facilities.

CASE IN POINT: MIDWESTERN HOSPITAL PREVENTS $750,000 ANNUAL OPERATIONAL DEFICIT THROUGH ITS SHELTER REFERRAL PROGRAM.

Due to an extremely high level of spouse abuse and its accompanying incidents of child abuse, one midwestern hospital faced some difficult decisions regarding its handling of these cases. By the conservative estimates of administrative personnel, the hospital was producing an operating deficit of almost $3,000 for every long-term care case involving an abuse victim. Because the caseload had climbed to over 250 annually, the financial toll imposed on the hospital was staggering.

Thanks to the creative thinking of its social service director, the hospital began to consult with the director of a privately operated shelter for battered women. This consultation ultimately lead to the transfer of abuse victims from the hospital to the shelter when their medical conditions were sufficiently improved to remove the need for further acute hospital care.

Operating through a program of volunteer people and a small staff of trained psychological counselors and social workers, the shelter began a rapid expansion process due to the major influx of new clients. Within one year, the paid staff had doubled and the volunteer staff had more than tripled. The shelter's net operating profit, to be reinvested into improvements, climbed by over 640 percent.

By removing this enormous caseload from the hospital's registry, the regularly recorded annual deficit of approximately *half a million dollars*, threatening the very existence of the hospital, was reversed. The hospital, three years after initiating the program, has turned the total hospital budget in the positive direction. Today, annual budgetary surplus exceeding $200,000 is expected as a regular occurrence.

This case history underscores the dramatic impact that an effective social services department can have on the financial outlook of a hospital. Making crucial connections with outside agencies or groups can often lead to major benefits for all concerned. Effectiveness, sympathetic service, and the financial stability of the hospital need not be mutually exclusive interests. As the preceding case history illustrates, it can be done to the mutual benefit of all concerned.

The Social Services Department and the Rape Victim

One of the most delicate areas involving the social services department surrounds the treatment of rape victims. Because rape is such an extremely "personal" crime, its victims are often shadows of their former personalities. Though many victims will attempt to put on a brave face in the presence of non-family people, the deep psychological pain inflicted by such brutality must be considered in any dealings with the victim.

Because rape victims are most often referred to the hospital by police agencies, a positive relationship between a hospital's social services department and local police agencies is essential to permit the most effective handling of these cases. Gaining access to pertinent information from police sources, sometimes the only reliable source for information in these cases, can often mean the difference between being able to assist the patient or watching helplessly as the patient crumbles into psychological chaos.

For larger hospitals, this social services role is particularly important. With a larger case load to be handled, the medical staffs tend to be more impersonal in their dealings with patients, often compounding the problems which the rape victim faces. Sympathetic listening and support from the social services staffer can help to cushion the impact of what may otherwise be an added psychological degradation of the patient, the examination process.

Though public information and awareness concerning hospital procedures surrounding rape cases has increased, making more women willing to report rape, this does *not* minimize the need for a psychological support structure to cope with rape's gruesome realities. No amount of public information can prepare the victim for the feelings of being violated and degraded through this insidious form of violence.

Because rape is a more prevalent crime in higher-population metropolitan areas, the larger hospitals should be placing a higher emphasis from social services in this area. Due to the diverse nature of victims' reactions, no ironclad procedural rules for handling rape cases are really possible. Sensitivity to the patient's needs, rather than "standard procedure", is really the best guide in these cases for the well-run hospital social services department.

Special Challenges for the Terminally Ill

No other event in the course of human experience has a more shattering effect on a family than death. Though the course of some illnesses, particularly in elderly patients, tends to prepare relatives for the patient's imminent passing from this life, the actual event is nonetheless an emotionally tearing experience for the survivors.

While some deaths are totally unpredictable, there is a considerable amount that can be done for relatives in cases where a patient's death is an expected result of the illness. Though the time span may involve only a matter of hours, not days, innovative ideas in social services programming can help to lessen the impact and produce important byproducts in the medical care process.

One example of beneficial results is in the tissue donor program. Though there has been a tremendous surge in the use of organ donor identification programs, many donations result from decisions made by relatives of the dying patient. Using innovative programs which emphasize emotional support for relatives in a time of personal crisis, this has eased the way to tissue donations after the patient's death. Though these psychological support programs were not initiated with any particularly mercenary intent, the end result has been a marked increase in tissue and organ availability for hospitals with the program.

As an example of how this works, let's take a look at one such program at a Western hospital.

CASE IN POINT: WESTERN HOSPITAL'S SPECIAL "INTENSIVE CARE FOR RELATIVES" PROGRAM REAPS MAJOR RESULTS.

Recognizing the need for an established program to meet the needs of relatives whose patients were in the intensive care unit, many on the brink of death, one western hospital decided to implement an Intensive Care for Relatives program as a special corollary to their regular intensive care unit activities. Normally composed of one chaplain and one social services staffer, this special team was called into action whenever a patient was admitted to the intensive care unit.

Serving as an informational conduit between the medical and nursing staffs and the patients' relatives, the special ICU team served to explain medical procedures to the relatives, freeing the doctors and nurses from this obligation. This provided more time to meet the physical needs of the patient, resulting in an improved survival rate due to greater ICU efficiency.

The nursing staff, relieved of these extra pressures, was better able to relate to relatives on a voluntary basis. Some nurses even reported a considerable increase in their job satisfaction resulting from this program.

For those patients whose death was a certainty, the work of the special ICU team was particularly valuable to the relatives. Through an intensive counseling process as the events were unfolding, relatives were able to increase their acceptance of the inevitable results. Because of this acceptance, the matter of tissue and organ donation could be discussed in a less emotionally charged atmosphere.

The end result of this process for this western hospital was an increase of over 10 percent in post-mortem tissue and organ donations.

There is little question as to the beneficial impact which this program can bring to a hospital. The only unmentioned benefit comes in the area of a hospital's public relations image. Because sympathetic care for the patient, as well as for the relatives, was made possible by this program, the amount of good will which the relatives will relay to the community—despite the adverse nature of the results of care (in death cases)—will be tremendous.

If your hospital does not currently have a program of this type in operation, these illustrated benefits should be sufficient to cause serious consideration of the program's potential. Maybe this idea is the "missing link" in your hospital's communications program with the community it serves.

Measuring the Results

As mentioned in the beginning of this chapter, any accurate assessment of social services department activities is rather difficult due to the intangible nature of its actions. One area of the operation is more easily analyzed. This is connected with the staff's interrelationship with their peers in other departments. The effectiveness of social services' connections with other parts of the hospital's staff is a crucial consideration in determining its overall effectiveness.

To determine "quality control" for this area, a considerable number of hospitals have instituted a form of peer review which is not restricted to the direct participants in social services department work. Through this method, a solid amount of "feedback" is made available to permit the social services director to analyze and quantify the department's capability in dealing with the hospital's ongoing caseload problems.

The peer review process, as adopted by these hospitals, incorporates representatives from administration, the nursing and medical staffs, and other hospital departments that have dealings with the social services sector. By not limiting input to the restrained confines of social service participants, a broader perspective is made possible.

To illustrate how this system works in actual practice, let's take a look at the peer review program as it was set into operation at one eastern hospital. Though no specific financial impact could be pinpointed through the procedure, the improved interdepartmental communication which resulted merits closer examination.

CASE IN POINT: EASTERN HOSPITAL SETS UP
SOCIAL SERVICES PEER REVIEW PROGRAM.

In an effort to assist the social services planning and implementation process, one eastern hospital decided to form a type of Peer Review Committee to study the activities of its department. Composed of representatives of every major hospital service and the head of the social services department, the committee met on a regular basis to discuss and study the problems common to their individual systems delivery functions. Because of their diverse backgrounds, the most common problem of peer review—the narrowness of viewpoint—was totally eliminated.

The committee has proved to be an excellent vehicle for developing new social services ideas to be implemented in the hospital, including a closer coordination with the community's clergy. As a direct result of this committee process, the improved coordination of activities resulted in an average 1.5 day reduction in the average stay for longer-term patients. Closer contact between social services and other departments meant that patient transitions were speeded up and general hospital efficiency was enhanced.

While direct cost estimates—particularly the savings caused by the program—might be hard to determine, internal conservative estimates have indicated a potential savings of 3 to 4 percent per patient stay.

While the results of this program, particularly from an administrative cost analytical viewpoint, might not be considered very dramatic, an intangible benefit of better staff morale and efficiency awareness would definitely have the effect of keeping social services staffers on their toes and aware of their impact on total hospital operations.

The greatest error in estimating a program's value is to view it singularly. Instead, we might suggest that the evaluation be made based on its incorporation into the total management program. A small benefit in one sector, multiplied with similar benefits in other sectors, can represent a major impact on the total financial picture for a hospital.

Hospital vs. Community Social Worker: The Difference

The hospital environment and the nature of its social services caseload provide a direct contrast by which to compare its functions to those of their counterparts in the community social services system. Because of the primary emphasis on health care aspects involved with his clients, the hospital social worker should concentrate attention and background on the medical aspects which contribute to the problems faced. Herein lies the major difference between the two major social service types, often a point which tends to disrupt the vital communications process between the two otherwise similar agencies.

By contrast, the community social worker views the field of endeavor in terms of the client's problems within the home and their relationships with the community at large. Though the problems of health must occasionally be drawn into the picture, the average community social worker may not have the medical background to address these issues. This is the primary reason that an effective liaison between the hospital social services department and its community counterpart is so important.

The viewpoint in these problems is the prime source for breakdowns in communication. Recognizing this factor is the most important first step in developing an effective working relationship between the two services. To help in minimizing this communications gap, some hospitals have attempted to recruit their hospital social services staff from the ranks of community social services, provided that they also have the necessary background to effectively address the problems which are singular to the hospital social service environment.

In almost every case where a hospital social services department was staffed with employees from a community service background, the problems of communication were virtually nonexistent. Direct knowledge of the other's viewpoint is the best assurance that a patient's best interests in transition from hospital to community will be served.

Closing Thoughts on the Social Services Process

Through this most directly people-oriented service that any hospital can provide, the health care system which your hospital institutes for community service is brought down to earth for easier public understanding. In personalizing the hospital's approach to its patients, the dehumanizing aspects which seem to be inherent in providing quality health care—particularly true in the larger, busier hospitals—can be markedly reduced.

Accurately described by one hospital social worker as "The People Connection," the great mission of hospital social services is to remove the remote character of the hospital health care process. Minimizing the psychological impact of hospitalization should be the foremost concern, aside from the transition coordination process, in social services department operations.

If this objective is achieved, despite the great difficulties in analyzing specifics of departmental operations, your hospital's department can be considered to be operating on a successful basis. Though the department is not immune from the budgetary concerns which plague other hospital departments, the relatively small percentage of the total operating budget which is normally devoted to social services should remove the major administration tendency to become "cents conscious" regarding this service.

More important than the monetary aspects of this service, the primary consideration (as emphasized earlier in this chapter) is the contribution social services makes to the smooth operations of the hospital. No department, regardless of its total operating budget or the nobleness of its purpose, should be permitted to be a detriment to the best interests of a hospital's continuing viability. Social services' activities are not immune from this rule.

This is the foremost criterion which you should be utilizing in your decisions affecting social services. If the department is making a visible contribution to your hospital's best interests, let the department have the limited autonomy needed to continue its activities efficiently.

By contrast, if the department shows itself to be detrimental, a critical appraisal of its activities is probably overdue. Administrative review, while seldom welcomed by social services directors, is the best way to assure that your hospital's fundamental management objectives are met now and in the future.

Coordinated planning steps for the multi-faceted rehabilitation services 18

WHEN A SEVERE ACCIDENT OR ILLNESS STRIKES, the predominant concern of the hospital's medical team has been the survival of the patient. This is as it should be. But the increased survival rate after these major illnesses or accidents, thanks mainly to advances in medical technology, has presented a mixed blessing to the surviving victim. He (or she) is confronted with what often proves to be a tandem obstacle, physical and/or psychological impairments.

This is where effective hospital rehabilitation services come into the picture. In order to be most effective in the total rehabilitation goal, the services should be organized to recognize that every major accident or illness has multiple victims. The person who sustains the injury is the most obvious victim. Less obviously involved, the relatives and the immediate family members are also "victims" in an indirect fashion. They must often make major adjustments in life style and attitude to accommodate the limitations of the stricken family member.

Because the rehabilitation services' objective is to return a patient to the most productive and full life that his impairments permit, incorporating the family into rehabilitation planning is a prerequisite to the patient's successful return to normal daily living. By maximum utilization of all facets of rehabilitation service, most patients can make a successful return to normal daily living.

The hospital's total rehabilitation program is actually a result of nine different services which have a direct impact on a patient's successful return from an illness or accident. The nine services involved are:

(1) The Medical Section
(2) The Physical Therapy Department
(3) The Occupational Therapy Department
(4) The Speech Therapy Department
(5) Psychological Services
(6) Social Services

211

  (7) Vocational Counseling
  (8) Prevocational Evaulation
  (9) Rehabilitation Nursing

  In order to gain a solid idea of the complexity of rehabilitation services, let's take a brief look at each of these nine sections to focus on their respective roles in the process.

(1) The Medical Section

  As mentioned in the beginning of this chapter, the primary objective is survival. The medical section of the process is initially concerned with this aspect of the patient's care. After the patient's initial critical phase has been concluded, the medical staff should consider the long-term impacts of the illness or accident, determining how much recovery can be expected and the methods by which this can be achieved.

  The rehabilitation process proceeds under the direction of the medical staff, with an ongoing process of monitoring conducted to be certain that no portions of the rehabilitation would trigger a relapse or complication of an existing problem. The medical staff also serves as the final judge of when a patient's expected recovery has been achieved, permitting the individual's release from further care.

(2) The Physical Therapy Department

  In cases of physical damage, this department is the most visible to patients and relatives alike in the total rehabilitation process. The objective in primary care hospitals is to enable an ambulatory or semi-ambulatory patient to be released to his home or to further care in rehabilitation nursing (discussed later).

  For illness-related cases, the CVA (stroke) being an excellent example, the department's objective is to gain movement and coordination in the affected limbs. Using a combination of passive and resistive exercises, patients can often gain a considerable portion of the functions which were lost.

  In accident cases, particularly where the loss of a limb was involved, the Physical Therapy Department's activities become meshed with those of a prosthetics service (an allied part of the department) to fit and aid the patient in adjusting to the artificial limb replacement. While this can be a lengthy process, mainly due to the complex combination of physical and psychological factors involved, the success rate in prosthetics has been phenomenal.

  Recent advances in Nerve-Response or Motor-Impulse propelled prosthetics have increased the role of muscle re-education therapy in the rehabilitation process. With these new advances, the limitations caused by the loss of a limb have been markedly curtailed, helping many patients to return to an almost completely normal life style after major accidents.

  As these technological advances continue, trends indicate that physical therapy services will continue to grow in importance. The science fiction of the past has become today's reality. The only real drawback to be considered is the cost/benefit balance. Capabilities will undoubtedly continue to expand. Unfortunately, the societal impact of technological costs may place a disproportionate squeeze on physical therapy services and unacceptably limit its potential.

(3) The Occupational Therapy Department

Redevelopment of physical skills is only one facet of a handicapped person's return to the normal flow of life. The impact of a disability, particularly for a younger person, may require a drastic reassessment of the work which can be expected. The total rehabilitation process must therefore include the direction of the redeveloped physical skills into constructive work.

During the training period in Occupational Therapy, the therapists can make some judgements as to what may be realistically expected from each patient. In doing this, the objective is to restore personal dignity to the patient and make him self-supporting again, whenever possible.

As an example, a person may have a substantial impairment of one hand. The occupational therapist, in conjunction with the patient, will attempt to develop activities which can be modified for satisfactory performance with one hand. Through diligent practice and the use of auxiliary assisting equipment, this person may be able to perform delicate handwork or operate a power tool with no difficulty. This assumes that no major impairment exists in the other hand.

Adaptability is the essence of this department's efforts with its patients. By successfully adapting daily activities to individual limitation, most people can lead fruitful, productive lives despite physical limitations. Making the most of available capacity is the ultimate goal for the occupational therapist.

(4) The Speech Therapy Department

As an aftereffect of some forms of brain injury, a person's ability to speak can be impaired. This can be the result of illness, such as a stroke or an encephalitic condition, or of an accident origin. In either case, the speech function can be rebuilt through persistent practice. This assumes, of course, that the entire speech control center of the brain has not been destroyed by the illness or accident involved.

Using a variety of techniques, which would include cadence adaptation and tongue guidance with wooden depressors, long tongue coordination can be redeveloped to restore intelligible speech. While temporary psychological problems often accompany speech difficulties, they usually lessen in direct proportion to the success of speech therapy treatments.

Most often, this area is neglected if the impairment is partial, favoring more intensive physical rehabilitation. Though this emphasis does meet society's need to return handicapped people quickly to the mainstream, the psychological limitations imposed by speech impairment could have an adverse impact on other aspects of the physical rehabilitation process.

(5) Psychological Services

In response to the mental anguish which often accompanies physical disability, many hospitals provide psychological support services to recovering patients to assist them in making the mental adjustment to their limitations. Using a combination of clergy services and professional counseling, the hospital's objective is to maintain the most positive mental outlook possible.

Some hospitals are fortunate is having members of the clergy trained in psychology who can combine spiritual and temporal counseling to troubled patients. If these clergymen happen to be the pastors or priests of a patient's congregation, the positive impact which the added familiarity brings can be a definite plus in the psychological improvement process.

This type of specialized counseling is usually limited to larger hospitals, particularly those that address regional rehabilitation needs, because the costs of full-time psychological counselors on staff can prove prohibitively expensive for smaller hospitals. Smaller facilities will use part-time visiting counselors, if any, to limit financial obligation.

For smaller hospitals, the most practical approach to acquiring these services is to develop a working agreement with a county mental health service agency or a similar group. Because there are usually such a small proportion of cases which really require the services of a trained psychologist or psychiatrist, the small hospital probably couldn't generate sufficient patient loads to warrant the salary retainer which these professionals would require.

(6) Social Services

The role of social services work in the rehabilitation process is basically one of easing the patient's transition from the hospital environment into the home or extended care nursing facility, depending on what the condition of the patient or the home environment might permit. Though we've already discussed the general overview of social service activities in Chapter 17, a quick re-cap of its specific function in the rehabilitation process is warranted.

In terms of a patient's family, the social service work is centered on helping relatives to make necessary adjustments to compensate for disabilities and to help arrange any needed equipment aids for the home, if they are desired. For cases which are marginally eligible for extended care status, the social services department can help the family to make an intelligent decision on the best course of action.

Hospital social services may also be able to acquire help form private and public agencies to assist patients and their families with equipment and other needed rehabilitation services. An example of this is possible referral to a local Easter Seal Society chapter or to the national organization for equipment assistance.

Regardless of the source, the main objective is to make the transition between two such diverse environments as hospital and home as smooth as possible. If that is accomplished effectively, the role of social services in the rehabilitation process will have been successfully completed.

(7) Vocational Counseling

For younger people handicapped by illness or accident, the transition from hospital to home life carries some additional problems. Earning a living and providing for a family can present major problems, particularly for the partially disabled person.

To meet this obvious need, vocational counseling is often instituted to help the person to choose work which he (or she) can perform within the new limitations imposed by the handicap. Portions, if not all, of this service can often be obtained through a government agency such as the Department of Vocational Rehabilitation.

This department's traditional emphasis has been on post-hospitalization training programs. After conducting an independent evaluation of a potential trainee, which includes a corroborating physical examination to confirm the nature and extent of any physical handicap, they sit down with the applicant and review potential vocational choices and available training programs.

At the time of this writing, considerable political pressure and public sentiment for federal budget cuts have jeopardized numerous federally based training programs. To date, this program has not seen any major reductions in funding and, considering the types of recipients involved, no such action would seem politically expedient at this time.

To cite some examples of their efforts, let's take a look at some successes they've been able to claim:

- Wisconsin double amputee had auto specially equipped and received training in computer programming techniques. Today, he is chief of computer operations for a manufacturing firm.
- Young California multiple sclerosis victim was trained in radio communications techniques. Today, he's a dispatcher for a metropolitan transit company.
- A Michigan cerebral palsy sufferer with controlled coordination in only one foot has been taught to use a computer with an interconnected voice synthesizer to substitute for his lack of speech. Using a stylus held between two toes of his right foot, this young man has progressed to developing his own original computer programs. Future plans are for him to establish his own independent programming business which he can operate from home.

These three people are examples of rehabilitation in beneficial action. Without added training and help from an outside source, these three—and thousands more with similar problems—could not be making the constructive contributions they're making today.

(8) Pre-vocational Evaluation

The evaluation of a handicapped person's capability is based primarily on the type of debilitating illness or accident suffered, the current state of recovery, and the amount of residual handicap which is expected to remain indefinitely. When these facts are combined with scientific aptitude and intelligence testing, trained counselors can make fairly accurate estimates of a person's abilities.

These results are then matched with the individual's areas of potential interest to arrive at a decision on vocational training. From the hospital's viewpoint, the main objective is to determine the patient's manual dexterity and capability to care for his (or her) own affairs. This dexterity analysis, in the larger picture, helps vocational analysts to pinpoint areas of potential weakness. The dexterity question, for example, would rule out small parts assembly if impairment was present.

This pre-vocational evaluation, most often conducted prior to release from a care or training program, is also a valuable tool for potential employers, helping them to decide if the applicant will effectively fit into their daily operations. The test results are often used as a selling tool to attempt placement of handicapped workers with potential employers.

(9) Rehabilitation Nursing

For the most persistent forms of illness or other handicap, the extended-care rehabilitation nursing program is the intermediate answer between acute-type hospital care and life at home. Though some hospitals accomplish patient transfers "on paper" to extended-care status, the most common method is to transfer the patient to an extended-care nursing home setting specifically designed to provide non-crisis care at lower costs.

Patients transferred to this status are judged not to require daily monitoring by a physician and have no acute illness other than their residual handicap. These patients are generally people who are unable to take care of themselves or have no one available for this purpose at home.

Because of the high demand for rehabilitation nursing services, there are often waiting lists for patients to enter these facilities. This factor can create a bureaucratic logjam within the acute care hospital. With a utilization standard which dictates patients' removal from the hospital—and no place to put them—a potential financial crisis is created.

The financial problem is triggered by insurance standards which halt payments if a patient is considered sufficiently recovered to no longer require acute care. If the patient can't be moved anywhere, who pays the bill? If the patient can't afford to pay, the hospital may get caught holding the bag.

Working as the Total Rehabilitation Team

Getting all of these diverse elements to work together efficiently can sometimes prove to be a major problem. If the available patient load makes it feasible for all services to be present in one facility, this can make a substantial contribution to total efficiency.

For smaller hospitals, the rehabilitation team is often limited to physical therapy services using a staff of two-year technicians with a registered physical therapist serving in a consulting capacity on one or two days per week. This expands to having a full-time registered therapist on duty in medium-size hospitals, along with a group of two-year technicians and other assistants to handle the non-technical aspects of physical therapy department activities.

Beyond the immediate needs of phsyical therapy to regain an ambulatory patient, many hospitals rely on a consulting service arrangement for other aspects of the rehabilitation service, if done at all. More often, the emphasis is on consolidating these services into a Regional Rehabilitation Service. Most experts believe that a population in excess of 100,000 is needed to generate sufficient patient load to warrant an extensive full-service rehabilitation program and facility.

Bringing all functions together helps a physician to more effectively monitor all facets of the rehabilitation program in which the patient needs help. Because the efforts are so intensive and multi-faceted, the patient benefits by reducing the time required for noticeable improvements. Faster rehabilitation often prevents major psychological problems and causes some fairly dramatic reductions in patient care costs.

The Regional Rehabilitation Center Concept

As mentioned earlier, a minimum population standard has generally been established to properly supply a rehabilitation center with sufficient patient traffic. For this reason, the regionalized rehabilitation center idea has caught on all over the United States. This is particularly true in the non-urban areas with lower population densities. The population criterion may be somewhat reduced in areas which have a higher proportion of older citizens, primarily because of the statistically higher probability of CVA cases.

The regional center is probably the only type of hospital, outside of the major metropolitan medical centers, where the full range of rehabilitation services can be offered on an economically viable basis. Most often, the cases referred to these centers involve people who are judged to have the greatest chance for an almost complete recovery. Those patients who are considered to have a lesser chance are more often placed in the care of an extended-care facility. If their case is judged, after reevaluation, to have changed markedly, they may also be eligible for the comprehensive rehabilitation center.

Because the nature of rehabilitation is frequently a long-term process, the design of rehabilitation centers should take psychological factors for patients into consideration. Prolonged separation from home and family seems to dictate that a rehabilitation facility's physical structure would assume as much of home-like features as can practically be incorporated without sacrificing the efficiency and success of the mission for which it was created. By maintaining a "residential" feeling in this design, situations can be created to stimulate feelings of independence, a vital portion of the rehabilitation process.

This design type also presents some solid financial benefits. Because of the comfortable environment, a facility like this becomes a chosen place for the rehabilitation process, virtually guaranteeing full occupancy and the financial viability needed to cope with economically erratic times. To underscore this point, let's take a look at the success of one such facility.

CASE IN POINT: NEW MIDWEST REHABILITATION FACILITY GROWTH TERMED PHENOMENAL. EXPANSION PLANNED AFTER ONLY ONE YEAR.

Thanks to expanded demand for services, one midwestern rehabilitation facility decided to expand its operations with the construction of a new 70,000 square foot facility costing slightly over $5,000,000. The innovative design of the building divides the center into four "courts" with a centralized covered courtyard for patients to gather and socialize.

Each room features an opening to an outdoor patio area for refreshments, getting outside fresh air and sunshine, and a barrier-free design which permits patients to go from the patios to other outdoor areas with the facility compound.

A section is provided outdoors for a raised garden which permits wheelchair-bound "green thumbs" to engage in their favorite pastime. Other similar activities are also designed on a raised platform system to make activities accessible to the facility's residents.

This activity-oriented design received high praise from the public. Within one year of its opening, all available beds in the facility have been filled, with a waiting list of new patients being kept to fill openings as they develop. This popularity has spurred plans to develop an expansion which would add 50 percent or more to its current size.

Scheduling: The Efficiency Key

Within the rehabilitation process, the major problem in coordinating the numerous facets is to assure efficient scheduling and avoid "cross-scheduling" which would put a patient in two different places at the same time. Developing a system which prevents this problem is the first priority in assuring that the rehabilitation program is operated in the most effective manner possible.

In determining scheduling, the most effective method appears to be the *priority system* which places patients in their most difficult therapy areas early in the day. For example, a patient who suffers from a major speech impairment that is more severe than the physical problems would be placed in the Speech Therapy unit first.

This system has two major benefits. First, the patient's performance in therapy is enhanced because he (or she) is fresh from a night's rest. Second, the department's more difficult cases are concentrated in the early parts of the day while the staff's ability to concentrate is at its peak. Later in the day, a decline of these factors might prove detrimental to both patient and staff.

Coordination of this system is best accomplished by having a centralized source to compare schedules and to coordinate traffic from patient care areas to the various therapy or rehabilitation consultation departments. The centralized source which appears to work best is to deposit patient therapy schedules with the facility's nursing staff.

As the coordinators of patient care, the nursing staff and its auxiliary aides are in the best position to help in implementing therapy schedules. Because they prepare patients for each new day, special emphasis can be placed on preparations for patients scheduled for therapy sessions early in the day.

By sharing more specific information with the nursing staff, the floor aide crew can be of even greater help in rehabilitation's efficiency objective. For example, if a patient is scheduled for a whirlpool treatment, the floor staff would not dress the patient in full pajamas or street clothing, opting instead for the common hospital gown which can be easily removed before entry into the whirlpool tub.

The shared information is actually the real key to making the scheduling system work. This also applies to the communications between individual portions of the rehabilitation system. By having a centralized "Master Schedule" rather than a group of individual schedules, these sources of misunderstanding can be eliminated. By maintaining the "team" psychological framework in all aspects of rehabilitation operations, the formation of this coordinated process will become a natural part of operating patterns.

Alternate Methods to Slash Costs

Due to the prolonged nature of the rehabilitation process in the majority of cases, the total cost becomes a major source of concern for the patient, his or her family, and to any insurance company involved in the reimbursement for services rendered. There is no way to deny the tremendous impact this factor has in any decisions made regarding prolonged care.

To restrain the costs of rehabilitation, the emphasis has been gradually switched from resident care in a rehabilitation facility to an outpatient mode whenever feasible. The feasibility of this idea is determined by the patient's physical condition as well as the availability of supervision and assistance in the home setting. The system ranges from the short-period rehabilitation and therapy session to the newest innovation in the development of rehabilitation planning, the Day Care Rehabilitation Center.

The Day Care Rehabilitation Center concept shows the greatest amount of promise for the future because it combines the intensive therapy regimen available in the resident care programs with the reduced cost factors commonly associated with the outpatient mode of operations. This combination represents an important advantage to all parties concerned with the rehabilitation process.

For the patient, the more intense rehabilitation therapy regimen means accelerated progress toward the ultimate level of recovery which is being sought. Maintaining the daily nature of therapy in an outpatient mode can keep the progress moving while, at the same time, offering some of the positive psychological benefits which are attained by permitting the patient to be in the home setting most of the time.

For the patient's family, the Day Care concept offers numerous advantages. Because the patient is only gone for the day, the family does not feel obligated to travel to visit their patient at the center. This continual traveling, conducted over a prolonged period, can have a very draining effect on the energies of family members. Another advantage is the freedom from patient care responsibilities. This factor alone can represent a major advantage, often helping to alleviate the financial impact which can result from the prolonged illness of a family member.

Insurance companies, and secondarily the family when insurance benefits run out, note the substantial reductions in costs which the Day Care Rehabilitation Center concept provides. The intensive day care rehabilitation program, as opposed to the resident care system, can represent a reduction of over 20 percent in the price tag charged for services rendered.

The day care system also represents a positive factor for the health care administrator, reducing the capital outlay requirements for new beds and other structural facilities. Though the transportation logistics for getting patients to the center on a daily basis can present a problem, these minor wrinkles can be fairly easily overcome if a degree of determination is shown in making the system work.

To underscore the enormous potential of this Day Care Rehabilitation Center concept, let's take a look at a system of this type that is currently in operation at an eastern hospital.

CASE IN POINT: EASTERN HOSPITAL USES DAY CARE CENTER TO REDUCE REHABILITATION PRICE TAG BY OVER 23 PERCENT.

When one eastern hospital decided to tackle the problem of rising costs for rehabilitation services, it came to the realization that the traditional residential care system was the real source of the cost control crisis. No amount of modification could change the fact that housing patients on a 24-hour-a-day basis was an expensive proposition. The only realistic alternative was to reduce the level of residential care at the facility.

This conclusion spawned the inception of the hospital's Day Care Rehabilitation program. The first problem confronted was the matter of transporting patients from their homes to the center on a daily basis. This problem was overcome by investing in a fleet of specially equipped buses to transport patients, mostly wheelchair-bound, to the facility.

After some initial problems with bus schedules were overcome, the program began to take off in a big way. Within four months, the Day Care Rehabilitation Center had reached its projected capacity with an opportunity to expand it further.

The cost differential of the established program, in comparison with the residential program, was substantial. Under the residential program, the daily cost was approximately $121.00 per day. Under the Day Care program, the cost amounted to only $93.00 per day. This represented a reduction of 23.1 percent through the innovative day care concept.

With an increasing public awareness concerning the inherent costs of health care delivery, cost reducing options such as the Day Care Rehabilitation Center concept are bound to gain increasing favor. The major point in favor of this plan, as illustrated by our case study, is the considerable reduction of costs.

Our objective in analyzing the possibilities for your rehabilitation services is to recognize the potential for alternative, non-traditional methods which can achieve the desired results. As with the Day Care Center idea, other alternatives should be measured by the same general criterion, meeting the primary departmental objectives at a reasonable cost.

If a serious intent to reduce costs is shown to insurance companies and hospital regulators, the major problems surrounding financial reimbursement to your hospital will be significantly minimized. From the administrative viewpoint, this is the greatest possible benefit which exploring alternatives can bring for your hospital.

Bringing the Pieces Together: Some Final Thoughts

The complete rehabilitation service, as we have discussed in this chapter, revolves around bringing all of the divergent services together into a cohesive whole. From the viewpoint of the patient and his or her family, the effectiveness of rehabilitation services is measured by only two criteria, the extent and rapidity of their loved one's recovery.

While this is natural, your measure should be of the more objective variety. Being able to achieve the maximum amount of results for the least possible total cost should be your primary objective. Because the very nature of rehabilitation has so many variables, including the distinct possibility that total recovery may not be possible for every patient, any analysis of departmental function based on success statistics could prove to be very misleading. For all too many patients, the best that can be expected is a partial recovery of the functions lost.

This fact leads to the greatest single problem in maintaining rehabilitation services at a high level—continued motivation of staff members. Because the tangible measure of success, particularly when dealing with elderly patients, can be so dismally poor, the process of maintaining staff morale in a seemingly losing battle can present a major test for administrative ability. If you succeed, the reward is a fine, efficiently operated rehabilitation service that any hospital would be proud to call its own. *

---

* See also ¶5501 *et seq.*, Prentice-Hall *Hospital Cost Management Service.*

Key elements of innovative hospital educational programming

19

As MEDICAL SCIENCE AND HOSPITAL HEALTH CARE technology continue their phenomenal growth, a concurrent need for expanded staff training for hospital employees and improved public understanding of health self-help developments become a dual challenge for a hospital's long-range educational programming. This double-faceted approach is the key to gaining maximum success in any hospital's plans for thorough education.

Staff members face an increasing problem of keeping up with the newest advances in their respective fields. The normal daily pressures of the job environment tend to inhibit independent study, making the problem of keeping modern standards in step with technological advances even more acute. Without the active participation and cooperation of the hospital, this is usually not possible.

A trend toward narrower definitions of professional activity, increased specialization, which has been started on a limited scale in some states, is opening new areas of opportunity for in-service training. With certification training programs being encouraged within the employee's own hospital (and this trend expanding to an increasing number of states), great new opportunities for professional growth, job satisfaction, and enhanced employee retention for participating facilities can be readily projected as a future benefit.

Educational program planners participating in these ambitious efforts are excited about the potential benefits to both the hospitals and the people they serve. The narrower definitions of professional activity, proponents assert, create a more thoroughly skilled staffer and improves the quality of health care being delivered to the public. As an example of this narrower professional definition, some states are now pushing for nursing certification in specific specialties as cardiac care and renal function nursing. This would put the certified nurses at a higher professional level and would give them preference in handling these specialized cases.

Program opponents argue that such narrow definitions would tend to increase costs for health care which are already being criticized in some circles as being excessive. While this might be a short-term result of the plan, the reverse argument that increased skill would result in greater efficiency and lower patient care costs would also be made. The long-range outlook would tend to validate the second argument far more than the first.

Regardless of which viewpoint a hospital's staff and administration might embrace, clear indications of in-hospital educational expansion are on the horizon. To meet this challenge and create favorable climate for employee retention, most hospitals will have little other choice than to develop and/or expand their in-house educational programming in the future.

On the community front, the hospital's educational efforts become a combination of public education and public relations as many facilities rush to embrace the growing trend toward childbirth classes for expectant parents, ostomy care classes, cardiopulmonary resuscitation (CPR) classes, and a host of other programs designed to make self-help and prevention gain wider public acceptance.

These public education programs have a tremendous public relations impact during a time when increased health care costs tend to make hospitals appear as the villain in every household's budgetary struggles. As the public perceives that a hospital is making substantial efforts to enhance their abilities to help themselves and reduce health care expenditures, greater acceptance of the prevailing costs when hospitalization is required is a natural byproduct.

During the course of this chapter, we will show how a hospital can initiate and develop these educational programs at minimal cost, often gaining access to vast material resources at no cost whatsoever. Though many of these sources might be considered of commercial origin, developing educational programming on the newest technological advances (these in particular) might best be done by utilizing the training materials provided by the manufacturers themselves. Because they are tailored to the specific products involved, developed by many of the same people involved in actual product development, their accuracy might be far more reliable than that of materials available through outside sources.

The non-product education materials are often available through similar sources, the result of very concerted public relations efforts by major corporations. Though the implied advertising tends to be woven into these materials, the major cost savings garnered through this method far offsets this minor disadvantage.

The In-service Training Program

Though much of the preliminary training for hospital staffers is frequently conducted in the university setting, the hospital's role in employee training has become an integral part of total professional development in many areas of hospital activity. Though nursing, the example cited earlier, is by no means the only area for this expanded training, it has become the most notable example of the principle in action.

The greatest emphasis for in-service training has recently been placed in the area of peripheral support services. The training of paramedics for ambulance service is a prime example of this trend. New or expanded requirements for professional competence in ambulance teams, while forcing out the funeral home business as the traditional provider of ambulance service as was common in the era leading into the 1960's, has resulted in vast improvements for ambulance service. Speed and capability of available service have both been enhanced by this development.

The hospital's role in this function has been to provide a training forum for these new auxiliaries to the health care process. Physicians, nurses, and other members of the hospital health care team have evolved into excellent instructors for this new service. As such, the availability of competent paramedics for community ambulance services, initially a major problem when the requirements were first mandated, has been vastly improved.

Organizing these educational programs, particularly in response to mandated requirements, requires a close coordination between administration, the departments most immediately affected, and the regulatory panels governing the program requirements. Because many of the rules and program ideas are so new, many hospitals hesitate to begin program development until the rules for their individual states are "firmed up" by the regulatory commissions.

While educational programming is usually developed by individual department chiefs to meet occupational needs, larger hospitals might find it advisable to consolidate educational programs under a single directorship. This position might be in the form of an assistant to the administrator or a director of educational programming. In either case, this director would be assigned the function of handling both internal staff training and the development of community education programs.

Coordination of efforts through this method would eliminate the possibility of training duplication, a very strong possibility in larger facilities with many small divisions within major medical services. Avoiding duplication is the surest way to keep the lid on expenses for staff education.

Smaller hospitals might consider the possibility of consolidating educational services to include the employees of several facilities in one program. By sharing costs, quality education for staffers is a possibility for even the smallest facility. The only possible trouble spot in this scenario is the cost for transportation of employees. If the training location is at a considerable distance, reimbursement of travel expenses in addition to wages paid during a time of lost productivity could wipe out any financial benefits that consolidation could bring.

These balance factors in determining the best route for pursuing employee education can create problems for some hospitals. Often, the best course of action in these marginal cases is to finance a single employee from a department to attend instruction seminars. In turn, this employee will bring back knowledge which can be passed on to his or her colleagues in the hospital.

The instruction seminar setup is of particular value because it creates a "faculty" for hospital training that is specifically trained in staff communications techniques, a solid advantage in any in-service training program. While this may require an initial investment to get things started, the long-term cost benefits in reduced travel expense and greater staff productivity will quickly repay the preliminary costs.

Based on these fundamentals, any hospital can develop an effective in-service training program, provided that sufficient administrative initiative exists to ferret out the opportunities for low-cost or free materials to help contain the costs.

The Hospital's Educational Budget

Due to the growing emphasis on in-service training, numerous avenues now exist to keep costs at a fairly reasonable level, often under $1,000 as the total start-up investment. This investment, when spread over a five to ten-year period (reflecting depreciation of equipment involved), makes the annual allocation of expenses quite small. In a growing number of cases, this initial investment represents the total expenditure involved in starting a hospital educational program.

Growing dependence on audio-visual material in the training process, reducing the amount of literature involved, is the greatest trend in limiting costs to the hospital. Using this technique, some hospitals have been able to acquire detailed training films, with the accompanying sound tracks, at absolutely no cost or the minimal expense of postage.

In other cases, films can be obtained for a small rental fee per film or as part of an annual rental fee for larger-scale usage. Though the trend toward videocassette recorder systems has caused a gradual shift in materials from movie film to videotape, there is still a vast reserve of movie film material available from many sources. The videocassette trend will, however, affect the course of future visual presentations. The declining cost of videotape as its use becomes more widespread will make it an attractive alternative to the current mode of movie visual production.

Though most analysts figure that videocassette recorder systems will decline in price as the market becomes more saturated with the units, the declining availability of new materials in standard movie mode would make the videotape system a fairly prudent investment right now. These videotape recorders, along with coordinated camera units now on the market, could prove to be the greatest single training aid for the hospital's educational program. (More about this a bit later.)

The complete videocassette equipment package, including the recorder/player and videotape camera, has been in the $2,000 to $3,000 price range, depending on the manufacturer involved. There are currently only two different setups on the market, the VHS and Beta systems. An important point to remember is that these are not interchangable, meaning that you can't play a VHS tape on a Beta machine or vice versa.

In deciding which type of system to purchase, the greatest consideration is the availability of materials for any given setup. Because the Beta system is the current dominant mode on the videocassette market, it's likely that most videotape programs are in this mode. This is not an endorsement of quality for the mode. It is merely a statement of current fact.

The Ultimate Training Aid

The videocassette system also represents a remarkable advance in training capability for the innovative education director. Using the videotape camera, students see themselves in action. This tends to make the process considerably more interesting than might otherwise be the case.

To fully appreciate the benefits this system can bring into the educational process, let's take a look at one successful program where the videocassette recorder and camera combo did the job more effectively than any other method.

**CASE IN POINT: MIDWESTERN HOSPITAL'S VCR SYSTEM
SPEEDS EMPLOYEE EDUCATION BY FIFTY PERCENT.**

Moving quickly to embrace the newest innovation of the Electronic Age, one midwestern hospital decided to incorporate the videocassette recorder and camera into their training equipment for staff education. Though the initial investment for new equipment was approximately $3,000, the hospital's education director felt it was a very wise investment.

"Thanks to this videotape system, we can reduce our staff training process time by at least 50 percent," the director stated. "By making full use of the system's potential, we have the most effective instructional tool ever created."

Here's how the system was used. The most prominent use was in the showing of previously produced instructional tapes. The secondary use, of equally importance, was the use of the unit's videotape camera. During practice exercises and emergency drills, one staff member filmed the action to be stored on videotape.

"We were able to offer a form of 'instant replay' on our activities during these practice sessions. Because the videotape was ready to be shown immediately, not needing film processing, we could review areas of problems that could develop into bad work habits," the education director said. "This type of thorough review meant that important portions of tasks could be learned, at minimum, the second time around by most students, cutting at least 50 percent from the learning time."

The preceding case example is a clear indication of the great potential which can be realized through the use of an innovative technique. Imaginative ideas can open the doors to such areas as in-house training films, low-cost training programs for small classes, and opportunities for training even a single employee.

Programming of this type is particularly important if staff turnover has been a problem at your hospital. Traditional training methods tend to be very expensive in the transition process. By developing and maintaining a small in-house library of training materials, the long-term cost of employee transition can be reduced by a considerable degree.

The "Satellite" Training Program

One of the greatest opportunities in hospital management to secure future staffing lies in a new innovation in health care education. As problems of cost continue to plague colleges and universities, they have become acutely aware of the resources around them. Their problems often prove to be a bonanza for the health care administrator in tune with the surrounding academic community.

Dramatic changes in university policy have enabled hospitals to create mutually beneficial programs, with the most dramatic advances coming in physician and nursing education. An effective partnership between a hospital and a college or university brings major benefits to both.

For the hospital, programs of this type have helped to alleviate staffing shortages by providing a pool of future employees. In providing a quality forum for their training, a hospital has an excellent opportunity to show its benefits to the participating students. Later, when these students graduate, recruitment by "the old Alma Mater" is received quite favorably. With all factors being equal, the hospital providing the training forum will often have the inside track in the graduate's choice of positions.

CASE IN POINT: MIDWESTERN EXTENDED-CARE HOSPITAL USES TRAINING PROGRAM TO SOLVE MAJOR NURSING SHORTAGE.

Faced with a major shortage of nursing staff, one midwestern extended-care hospital decided to meet the challenge head-on by developing a partnership with a nearby university nursing program. As the program began, the hospital had only 55 percent of the normal contingent of nurses considered to be required for optimum operation.

Because the hospital dealt exclusively with long-term patients, the vast majority being elderly, most nursing school graduates had not seriously considered employment at such a facility. Thanks to the exposure offered in the training program, this attitude began to reflect major changes.

When the first graduating class of 22 Licensed Practical Nurses completed training, the hospital was able to retain ten as regular members of the nursing staff. This trend continued until, five years after the program was initiated, the entire nursing shortage was wiped out.

"We're very pleased with the nurse training program and our participation in it," the hospital's administrator stated. "We now have enough suitable applicants to fill our normal attrition rate and avoid the nursing shortages experienced in the past."

This case history reflects only the tip of the iceberg regarding potential satellite training benefits. This also extends to the area of physician training and hospital internship or residency programs. Similar retention rates are being recorded in many areas of the country. This normal trend, provided that the training experience was a positive one, has occurred in almost every hospital that has participated in these programs.

Though Community Tuition Grant systems, programs which provide tuition money in exchange for a commitment to practice in a community for a set number of years, have had a considerable effect on satellite programs; the retention rate of quality training programs has remained sufficiently high to maintain their status as first-class recruitment tools.

Expanding the Educational Horizons

The establishment of quality educational resources within the hospital for initial training purposes is really only the beginning of its potential. Most professionals welcome the opportunity to expand their knowledge and skills beyond the minimum requirements set out to gain their degrees. This desire gives the educationally oriented hospital an excellent opportunity to create a favorable atmosphere for staff retention as well as to enhance the quality of services rendered.

One of the best ideas in this area for any hospital is the establishment of a small, but quality, medical library. Quite often, members of the medical staff will readily contribute books and professional journals as the "seed" from which the facility can grow. Though money is often a major consideration, subscriptions to the major professional journals, particularly those which cover medical or surgical specialties offered by the hospital, can be an excellent first step. Reference books on surgical anatomy, medical texts, and some pharmaceutical manuals warrant space in the library.

Another area for consideration in the library is coverage of nursing services. Like the physicians, a hospital's nursing staff can benefit immensely by having solid reference materials available to provide quick refresher courses in techniques which are not frequently used. Occasionally, a specialized case may arrive at the hospital, requiring additional procedural information. Maintaining information of this type is certain to have a major beneficial effect on the quality of care which a patient can expect.

If funding permits, the library might also consider including reference manuals written by medical or surgical specialists to give a hospital's general practitioners expanded knowledge in dealing with the more complex cases they are forced to confront. By making materials of this type available to the staff, the quest for improved knowledge and skills can continue on an informal basis with very beneficial results.

One major benefit of an enhanced library system is the greater likelihood of medical staff retention. In having an environment that fosters intellectual expansion, a hospital shows real concern for the needed professional growth which staff members recognize as the lifeblood of their work.

While it is quite possible to spend a hospital "book broke" in establishing a medical library, the beginnngs can be relatively modest. With annual budgetary allotments geared for its expansion, the hospital's library can quickly prove to be an intellectual center of activity for many of the hospital's medical and nursing staffers. By failing to capitalize on this potential a hospital can effectively limit its growth potential and discourage the natural process which prevents a facility's stagnation and eventual demise.

If your hospital does not presently have a medical library, we recommend that you consider implementing a library plan as soon as it is financially feasible. If you already have a library in place, be certain to review its needs periodically. The value of a library is directly proportional to the immediacy of its contents. When materials are hopelessly outdated for staff use, the library's value declines rapidly.

With only a little bit of administrative foresight, a hospital's medical library can prove to be one of the best behind-the-scenes educational programs that a hospital can offer its staff.

The Community Connection

The hospital's role in community health education has been a growing trend during the past decade. Largely based on a new awareness of the "prevention ethic," an increasing number of hospitals have begun to institute in-hospital community education courses, with particular concentration on courses for specialized conditions.

As a direct example, many hospitals now offer the popular concept of natural childbirth within the educational program of childbirth training (often referred to as the Lamaze Method). The childbirth classes are probably the largest single hospital education sector that is actively pursued in American hospitals today.

The emphasis in this class, along with other such hospital-oriented courses, is to remove some of the natural apprehensions which patients face in the hospital health care process. Knowing what can be expected, patients and their relatives will know when outside help is needed. This often prevents panic, a somewhat natural aftermath of a potential emergency situation.

In the case of CPR training, hospital education can actually be a lifesaving service to the community. This program, with active involvement from the community, can mean that a person skilled in CPR can be available within minutes for almost every cardiac emergency case. These precious minutes can mean the difference between death, or life as a brain-damaged invalid, and the return to a productive and useful life.

CASE IN POINT: SEATTLE'S COMMUNITY CARDIAC EDUCATION PROGRAM GAINS MAJOR RESULTS.

In the early 1970's, Seattle recognized the major community problem created by coronary disease. This threat to public health demanded that a great community effort be undertaken to combat the devastation which could result.

With the cooperation of doctors, nurses, and area paramedics, a comprehensive educational program was initiated to bring the lifesaving CPR message to the community. Using the resources of hospitals and the public school system, courses were soon offered to adults and children alike, bringing this life-sustaining art to everyone's attention.

Because of this intensive effort, Seattle is now considered the safest place in America to have a heart attack. Depending on which expert's statistics one wishes to believe, one in four to one in three of Seattle's residents is now capable of administering CPR and saving a heart attack victim from imminent death.

This case study reflects only a beginning for hospital education program. Combining the resources of a hospital with other community resources, as was done in Seattle, can vastly improve health care for everyone.

Hospital educational programs also address such specialized areas as ostomy care. In the case of ostomy care, the program is a combination of technical assistance and psychological support for patients. Due to the traumatic nature of ostomy surgery, patients often require psychological counseling and support to deal with the daily routines that ostomy surgery imposes on daily life.

Though patients can often lead reasonably happy and productive lives despite these surgical alterations, continuing psychological support systems (often using patients who have successfully dealt with the problem to counsel newcomers) are an integral part of a hospital's post-care efforts with patients.

Expanded External Resources and Their Costs

For many hospitals, the prospect of maintaining a large stock of informational films and materials can represent a prohibitive cost. To combat this problem, development of regionalized information centers has become an increasing trend throughout the United States. Using the shared-cost approach, these centers can offer a much larger selection of materials to participating hospitals than any facility could feasibly maintain individually.

CASE IN POINT: WESTERN PROGRAM OFFERS LOW COST ANNUAL EDUCATIONAL RESOURCE PROGRAM.

To address the educational needs of many western hospitals, one firm offers a large selection of videocassette programs, slide/tape combination presentations, and audio-tape recordings for hospital educational use.

For the current annual fee of $400, a hospital can borrow any two of these programs at one time for use as an educational tool for its staffers or as an "extension education"-type program. Under the prescribed-period loan program, the material is used for a predetermined period and then returned to its source.

Considering that many of these programs would cost from $75 to a top figure of approximately $150, this annual-fee program has been a clearly valuable cost-cutter for participating hospitals. Using an extensive educational program, a hospital could easily save $3,000 to $7,000 annually through this rental program.

This illustrated program is one of several similar program concepts currently being offered on a regional basis around the United States. Similar cost savings are offered by most of these programs. If you're currently hesitant about initiating an education program for your hospital, this idea may be just the key to making an extensive educational program economically feasible.

Hospital Education: Some Closing Thoughts

During the course of this chapter, we've attempted to give a preliminary overview of the hospital education topic. Admittedly, the information given here is not all-inclusive. An entire book could conceivably be written on the subject.

More important, we've attempted to give you the "germ for thought" which is necessary before meaningful innovation and advancement can take place. Quite often, limitations in assessing the education program's potential contribution to the hospital can be the greatest cause for its failure.

For most such programs, the question is not one of absolute failure. Rather, they tend to limp along at a slow pace which does not make the effective additional contributions to the hospital management picture.

Educational programming can be a vital contributor to the future success of any hospital. Professional advancement through education is often the key element which enables a hospital to attract top-flight people to its staff. The availability of educational resources can easily make the difference between having the best possible professional staffer and settling for an "also-ran" from the profession's ranks.

Public relations, always a matter of major concern for most hospitals, is also affected positively by an effective educational program. A hospital that is publicly perceived as having sufficient community concern to educate its citizenry will surely generate greater support for its health program needs than a facility that is apparently indifferent to the community it serves.

From every viewpoint, hospital educational programming is the best key to molding the bond between the administration and its staff. The same principle applies to its relationship with the community.

Organize it! Aggressively promote its welfare! Those are the two keys to making hospital education a viable force in your community. If you accomplish this, your hospital will lay the foundation for success in every area of its designated health care missions.

Successful utilization plans for volunteer services 20

VOLUNTEER SERVICES, the hospital's version of the proverbial free lunch, is one of the most vital areas of concern for most administrators. Particularly for the Community Hospital, the central core of dedicated volunteers serves to bridge the gap between patient needs and the financial realities of hospital management.

In addition, volunteer services have been known to provide valuable fund-raising assistance for the hospital, enabling the purchase of equipment or financing treatment programs that might otherwise be unattainable.

The area of volunteer services is a fairly broad based one, ranging from volunteer ambulance drivers and attendants within the community to the women of the Hospital Guild who operate little gift shops within the hospital for the benefit of different internal projects. This also would include help for inpatient care, with volunteer aids and the Red Cross program for orienting high school students to the needs and regimen of nursing (commonly referred to as the "Candy Striper" program).

Also included in this large list of community volunteers is the local clergy, helping the hospital to meet the spiritual needs of its patients. Through a well-coordinated chaplaincy program, these vital services can be delivered at little or no cost to the hospital. Though no specific wages are paid for these services, the minor cost involved is concerned with administrative and staff time in coordinating these volunteer activities.

This coordination is a vital part of the management picture, making certain that none of the volunteer activities directly conflicts with the primary activities of the hospital's mission to the public. In most cases, these volunteer services are designed to meet personal patient needs, rather than the financial needs of the hospital.

Bringing together an effective and successful volunteer program can prove to be a challenging, but very rewarding, aspect of your administrative activities. The major improvements in patient morale that often accompany the efforts of volunteers can serve as an excellent tonic for patients whose major impediment to recovery is their attitude toward hospitalization.

The Hospital Guild

A major contributing element in the hospital volunteer spectrum is the Hospital Guild structure within each facility. As a group of dedicated volunteers, their time and talents can be a major source of extra revenue for necessary hospital projects that might otherwise be neglected due to financial constraints.

As mentioned in the beginning of this chapter, one of the most common projects that might come under the Guild's jurisdiction would be the hospital's Gift Shop. This area provides for the sale of small items, often coming in as contributions from Guild members, which are sold to patients and their visitors to raise funds. Other possible methods which Guilds might utilize would include bake sales, raffles, bingo games (where legal), and other assorted methods of fund-raising.

The effectiveness of Hospital Guild activities has been so broadly recognized that formation of Guilds has been encouraged in almost every hospital service area in the nation. Each year, the list of active Guilds grows in direct proportion to the needs exhibited by the benefiting hospitals.

They remain effective because of the relatively high priority that the public places on the needs of the hospital. Considered as the "painless" method of attaining the financial goals for special hospital projects, the growth of Guild-generated revenues has historically been able to keep pace with inflationary pressures, without suffering proportional declines during difficult national economic trends. This fact has made Guild activities one of the most stable sources of revenue that hospitals depend on.

The level of volunteer support for hospital activities might best be illustrated by the following account of a successful volunteer program in an eastern Pennsylvania hospital.

A CASE IN POINT: VOLUNTEERS SUPPORT HOSPITAL'S CANCER TREATMENT PROGRAM.

For one eastern Pennsylvania hospital, the force of volunteer commitment and its effects will never be underestimated. Through a variety of fund-raising efforts sponsored by the Hospital Guild, this hospital was able to successfully launch a cancer treatment center within its confines.

The monumental nature of this volunteer effort can only be appreciated when you consider that the entire $85,000+ budget for operating the program annually is being raised through the volunteer community efforts spearheaded and sponsored by the hospital's active and effective Guild activities.

That $85,000 figure is a very impressive one to be attributed to direct volunteer efforts. The major point to remember is that this commmunity involvement became possible because concerned citizens were inspired by an effective hospital administrator. Similar inspiration could come from you to the community your hospital serves.

Recruiting Hospital Volunteers

Establishing an effective network of hospital volunteers is probably the best possible example of effective hospital public relations in action. The image which each hospital projects to the community will have a substantial impact on the number of volunteers who will be made available for various hospital projects.

The first element you should consider is the potential sources of volunteer help within your community. Explore the possible liaisons which you could establish with local established service organizations within your community. Church groups, fraternal organizations, high school students' organizations, college groups, and similar organizations can prove to be an excellent source of volunteer help for any hospital.

The second element in the recruiting process is the effective motivation of potential recruits to volunteer their time. Because monetary reward is not the motivating factor, you must rely on psychological "keys" to get your people moving.

The most common motivation is community pride. Every citizen wants to see top-notch facilities within his community. That element of civic pride can be the greatest motivational factor working for you in this recruiting effort.

Finding Motivational Keys

Unlike the employees of your hospital, whose tangible monetary gain serves as a motivating factor, the volunteers serving your hospital must be motivated by other techniques. In developing your volunteer program, you should place considerable emphasis on ideas for gaining top performance.

In the area of fund-raising activities, conducting effective volunteer activities can literally mean a "life and death" difference for some major hospital programs. The case of the cancer treatment program was a prime example.

One excellent method which has been successfully utilized revolves around the "Award Concept," i.e., providing recognition for the top fund-raising group or individual efforts which have been outstanding. This recognition can vary from an honorable mention in the local newspaper to a lapel pin award or a small plaque which recognizes exceptional volunteer efforts.

To underscore the effectiveness of some tested methods, let's take a brief glimpse at some solid ideas in action.

CASE #1: HOSPITAL ENDS CRISIS
OF VOLUNTEER SHORTAGE.

For over 20 years, one midwest hospital operated a very loose coalition of volunteer activities designed to provide extra patient services and enhance the atmosphere of the hospital. While the objective of the program was solid, the staffing levels for the volunteer group were chronically low. To aggravate the problem, participation was slowly declining to the point of making the program totally ineffective in meeting hospital needs.

With the decline continuing, and few new volunteers appearing to replace those who were leaving, the administrator launched a program which would encourage and recognize longevity in the volunteer program. In addition to this, he also initiated a recognition program for recruiting efforts made by individual volunteers from the existing organization.

After six months, the administrator organized a Hospital Volunteer Recognition Dinner which was covered by the local television and radio stations, augmented by newspaper coverage. At this recognition dinner, an assortment of lapel pins honoring various lengths of service were given to hospital volunteers. Additionally, the Annual Hospital Volunteer Recruitment Award plaque was unveiled. The name of the year's leading recruiter would be engraved on the plaque to be displayed in the hospital lobby.

What were the results of this program? Within three years, waiting lists had to be established for volunteers awaiting functions which they might be able to join. During this period, the level of volunteer support activities within the hospital have grown by 150 percent. Unofficial estimates place the value of services rendered at over $200,000 annually, not counting the funds raised to support valuable hospital activities.

The cost budgeted for recognition activities has ranged from $750 to $1,000 a year for the program. That's a return of one dollar for every *half cent* invested by the hospital. No other investment made by the hospital has ever reaped such rich dividends.

CASE #2: HOSPITAL AND SCHOOL UNITE FOR SUCCESSFUL "RADIO-THON" FUND RAISING EVENT.

Facing the need to raise a considerable amount of money in a short period to be eligible for a substantial government grant, a hospital in the south central states ran a brief news item in the local newspaper describing its problem and asking for suggestions from the community on ways to solve it.

The high school, sponsoring a class in radio arts and sciences, proved to be the key to solving the problem. The radio arts class took the problem as their class project.

After first contacting the hospital's administrator to gain his approval, the class approached the owners of an all-night radio station in the area to outline their proposal. Their idea was to conduct a 16-hour All Night Hospital Benefit Radio-thon with listeners calling in their pledges of monetary contributions for the hospital's project.

With radio station approval, the students went to work in organizing their program for the event. The efforts proved to be an overwhelming success. The metropolitan residents responded enthusiastically, at an average rate of $10,000 an hour, raising over $160,000 for the hospital.

Needing only $150,000 to serve as the local share of the government grant, the hospital used the additional $10,000 to offer a scholarship to a local student who had gained acceptance by a recognized medical school.

By any standards, the volunteer effort was a resounding success. The hospital's costs for the entire program were limited to minor supervisory time provided by the administrator. No financial outlay was required.

The second case example clearly illustrates a sound axiom of effective motivation—directly tying a volunteer's current interests into the activities that will benefit the hospital. If you are able to effectively correlate the activities which the volunteer currently has with your hospital's interests, you stand a greater chance of gaining a willing volunteer.

For example, you might be able to recruit a local artist to paint a small landscape picture to beautify a patient lounge area. A talented newcomer in the field might be your best bet for this attempt. Seeking an opportunity to gain public display for his (or her) work, he may jump at the chance to have his work hanging in an area where fairly large numbers of people might gather.

These are merely ideas from which you can develop a springboard to effective coordination of volunteer activities. The most important point to remember is to connect talents with available jobs. This connection will usually yield the greatest dividends for your hospital.

Coordinating Volunteer Activities

In order to gain maximum benefit from volunteer participation in hospital activities, efforts should be made to coordinate these activities with those of the paid staff of the hospital. Definite rules regarding volunteer functions must be drawn up to avoid the potential of chaos in required medico-clinical activities.

Your function, from the administrative viewpoint, is to set up solid guidelines which are mutually acceptable to both staff and volunteers. There is a definite need for an open line of communication between your office and the staff in guideline development. Because each hospital is as individual as a human fingerprint, it would probably be unwise for this book to set out specific "must do" imperatives for these guidelines.

However, there are specific areas in which some potential conflicts could arise. Preventing these problems can be the best avenue to create a major success in your volunteer programming.

For the sake of reference, here are a few potential problem areas which you should avoid:

(1) Volunteer activities should never be permitted to interfere directly with clinical activities.
(2) All patient care volunteers should be advised of the confidentiality which must be provided for all information regarding medical conditions. (In colloquial terms, don't go blabbing about someone else's illness. No gossip spreading!)
(3) For appropriate coordination with regular departmental activities, volunteers should be under the direct supervision of the department head whose daily employment activities are most closely affected by the volunteers' actions. (Unsupervised activities could be a source of administrative chaos.)

The essence of the administrative problem here, as in almost every other area mentioned in this book, is the communications factor. Keeping the free flow of information moving between your office and the volunteer help which serves your hospital will help to keep everyone's efforts coordinated toward the common goal of your administration.

The Chaplaincy

Aside from the immediate physical needs of your hospital's patients, another equally important sector of their care, their spiritual needs, should be effectively addressed by administrative policy.

Most community nonsectarian hospitals have developed a standing policy regarding open access of the clergy to members of their respective congregations when they are hospitalized. This essential element of hospital public relations has been a tradition practiced by hospitals for many decades. No specific reasons have ever been presented, from a management viewpoint, that would warrant major changes in this policy.

Daily implementation of this general objective can, however, be somewhat tricky. As in the case of other hospital volunteers, the need to avoid impediments to the hospital's primary clinical mission applies equally to members of the community's clergy.

Your office should make every effort to form an effective communications link between the hospital and the clergy, conducting regular meetings (or as mutually agreed upon) to discuss the needs and problems of the clergy in administering to the spiritual needs of the patients.

Traditionally, very few standing restrictions are placed on chaplaincy activities within the hospital. Though the clergy are required to observe any restrictions imposed by hospital conditions (i.e., quarantine and standard isolation procedures, etc.), ministers are usually permitted to enter and leave the hospital as they see fit, regardless of the hour involved.

The only standing restriction usually placed on the clergy is to avoid the tendency to "evangelize" (convert) other patients, non-members of their congregations. These non-member patients might consider these clergy activities to be a form of psychological harassment that could have an adverse effect on the high posture of public relations which your hospital would wish to maintain.

Chaplaincy Procedures

To insure that this last admonition is observed, most hospitals maintain a registry of patients according to religious affiliation. This registry is available for inspection at the hospital's business office.

Information for this registry comes from the standard question maintained in the regular admission procedures for new patients. When an incoming patient indicates his religious preference, it is listed in the patient registry.

During their periodic visits to the hospital, each member of the clergy inspects the lists provided to pick up the names of patients who belong to their church. These visits serve as a vital link for the patients, particularly for those who have been hospitalized for a prolonged period.

In cases involving critically ill patients, almost all hospitals open their doors to clergymen to visit the patients, even during the middle of the night (if the prevailing conditions indicate this might be advisable).

In some hospitals featuring a nondenominational chapel, local clergy may periodically conduct services for the semi-ambulatory patients who can be brought into the chapel. Hospitals with extended-care patients will often use this method as a means of boosting patient morale, offering a measure of normality to the lives of people who have been confined away from the mainstream of public life for long periods.

Every hospital, in developing its patient policies and public relations, has an obligation to maintain the religious well-being of its patients as well as their physical health. Because the psychological health of a patient has such a great impact on recovery progress, most physicians and administrators readily agree that the community's clergy play a vital role in the medical recovery process.

Hospital Volunteers: Some Final Thoughts

As we stated in the opening of this chapter, the hospital's volunteer program plays a vital role in the total picture of the quality and quantity of care which any hospital can deliver to the public. The real key, however, in the volunteer picture is its ability to improve the quality of life, to add the personal touch which can make a make a major difference.

The volunteers offer a commodity which can be more precious than any money could ever be. They are offering their time. What makes it more meaningful is that they do it because they *really care*. Because they are not being paid for their services, patients recognize that they are there because someone needs them. The volunteers reach out to touch the lives of those for whom there may be no one else left in this world.

These caring people separate the hospital from the status of a mere institution, giving it a humanity which might not be possible by any other means. They permit the hospital to fulfill the final part of their mission, being the "helping hand" that really counts in a time of combined phsyical and emotional stress.

Look around you today. Consider the many services which these people bring to your hospital. Then think about what conditions might be like without them. The difference you would see speaks volumes for the value of the volunteers who serve in hospitals across the United States today.

Those volunteers really do count! Let them know it! That message will make their performance even greater to the future best interests of your hospital.

Expand your hospital's revenue base with innovative management techniques

IS THE POTENTIAL FOR YOUR HOSPITAL'S REVENUE BASE a considerable distance from its ultimate realization? You may have only "scratched the surface" of the hospital-tested techniques you might implement to gain maximum utilization and revenue production from your current facilities.

Challenging statement? Perhaps! But it was intended to be precisely that. You may recall, from an earlier chapter, our discussion of the hospital laundry which took in the work from other hospitals. This idea was merely a proverbial drop in the bucket to the total potential which your hospital might realize, provided that you begin, right now, to thoroughly assess the current situation of your hospital.

In this chapter, our main objective will be to expand your view of your total operations picture, to enhance your vision of the possibilities contained within the walls of your hospital, and to capitalize on the new horizons which you will come to recognize.

Dropping Departmental Stereotypes

The first step in the truly innovative program is banish forever the notion that certain departments must be limited to the narrow scope of activities which might be generated within your hospital.

The acknowledged source of most, if not all, financial problems within hospitals has chronically proven to be the under-utilization of staff. While most departments have minimum staffing requirements to meet usual peak period workloads, these so-called peak periods are not that frequent or prolonged. This leaves each supervisor with the problem of low productivity due to overstaffing during the non-peak periods.

This fact opens the door to innovative solutions which can effectively expand departmental and hospital revenue dramatically. The essence of the proposed solutions comes from seeking ways to sell these services (performed during non-peak periods) to outside sources, generating extra revenues for the hospital.

Every method which you can come up with that will bring in extra money for the hospital will enhance the financial outlook of your hospital. Occasionally, this "extra" money can literally make the difference between a financially sound institution and one which is heading for financial collapse.

Selling the Service

While most professionals, particularly those centered in health care delivery services, are concerned with the ethical considerations involved in expanding different aspects of their services, this concern is generally being outweighed by the formidable requirements of increasing available revenues. In realistic terms, the items and methods which will be proposed here do not carry potential ethics considerations.

With the possible exception of one item which may be prohibited in a few states (we'll flag the item for special attention and discussion), the rest of the techniques for expanding hospital income carry no legal repercussions whatsoever.

The point that should be emphasized is to make every effort to find all conceivable outlets for the unused service time that is usually available in almost all hospitals. This sales push can result in major monetary gains, as several of the upcoming examples will clearly show.

Dealing in Specifics

Up to this point, we've discussed the revenue expansion theory in rather general terms. To illustrate how this idea can gain practical application within *your* hospital, let's take several departmental examples and indicate areas which you might be able to sell to outside revenue sources, enhancing your financial outlook.

(1) The Business Office

With major advancements being made in office technology, productivity potentials have been increased dramatically. This has opened the door for major opportunities for the creative administrator to expand hospital income from this source.

The advances made in computer technology have been in the forefront of this major surge in income potential. Utilizing computers has enabled hospitals to consider expanding their services to the community, outside of the basic health care mission.

CASE IN POINT: A HOSPITAL FINANCES A COMPUTER SYSTEM BY SUBLETTING BUSINESS SERVICES.

With the installation of a medium-size computer in their business office, one eastern hospital found that its internal hospital business was being conducted in less than half the time which was previously required to complete the same tasks.

Faced with the choices of expanding the availability workload or furloughing a major portion of their business office staff, this hospital's administrator decided to begin offering "Computer Time" to local small businessmen. For a nominal fee, the hospital's computer would handle the accounts receivable and send out bills as the recorded accounts warranted.

The response to this idea was substantial from the business community. Thanks to this innovative approach, an additional $100,000+ annually was brought into the hospital. An additional benefit was that none of the existing business office personnel were required to be furloughed. The hospital and its staff benefited equally from this approach to business management.

The financial return realized by this hospital, thanks to its external marketing program, was in addition to the savings in labor and materials costs for the operation of hospital accounting practices. With the influx of additional cash, similar systems in other hospitals could become self-sufficient rather quickly, usually paying for themselves in slightly over a year.

The use of innovative utilization ideas has opened the door to the Computer Age for this hospital. It could do the same for your hospital, or enhance the profitability of your existing systems. Think about it! This could be the "ticket" for you. *

(2) Hospital Communications

Thanks to the newest in videotape technology, the concept of an internal educational broadcasting system to present educational films to patients through a standard television installation has become a reality.

The only hindrance to this bright scenario has been the potential revenue source to offer a tangible payback for the system. Let's take a look at how one hospital tackled the problem and found the solution.

CASE IN POINT: BINGO GAME PAYS THE WAY FOR ADVANCED HOSPITAL TELEVISION.

With an acknowledged need for an effective patient educational "vehicle" that required small staffing to operate, one eastern hospital settled on the idea of installing a videotape machine that could be piped into patients' rooms through an unused channel in the remote control televisions which were already installed.

The only major drawback was the inherent costs of setting up the system. The videotape machine alone cost over $1,000. The means to get the signal into the televisions added considerably to this price tag.

Using some unorthodox planning ideas, the hospital staff used the camera which was part of the unit to set up their own Bingo game show for the patients. For a small fee, patients could participate in the daily bingo game being broadcast into the rooms. The first prize was a $25 savings bond.

Patient reaction and participation were quite favorable. As a result of this ongoing fund program, the hospital was able to regain its investment in less than two years. The cost of patient information programming has been absorbed by the proceeds from this game show.

---

* See also ¶3901 *et seq.,* Prentice-Hall *Hospital Cost Management Service.*

Thanks to this innovative programming, vital patient educational assistance can be offered with *no increase* in hospital costs and *no resulting increase in hospital charges* to cover the educational program.

This idea clearly illustrates that employing unusual techniques can sometimes result in substantial rewards for the hospital. We must caution you, however, to check local and state regulations before initiating this particular type of program. Your state might require a low-cost annual permit to operate a Bingo game. This cost should not be of major significance, particularly if you emphasize the non-profit nature of the idea to the officials you contact.

(3) Laboratory Innovations

One source of extra hospital revenue often overlooked by hospital administrators is the Laboratory. Here, as in other areas of the hospital, non-peak periods can rob the hospital of essential productivity that could be a major source of needed cash flow.

The essential element is to find productive ways to fill the non-peak periods. Some potential solutions that might be considered would be to solicit business from the Public Health Service, local physicians not practicing within your hospital, and other similar professional areas which require laboratory services.

One innovative idea (here's that *flag* item!) that might be instituted within your hospital's lab is to run tests for area veterinarians. The reasons that this could present a regulatory problem stem from prohibitions in some areas against testing animal specimens in the same facilities used for testing human specimens. While this regulatory prohibition is not, to our knowledge, widespread, you might find it advisable to check with state licensing autorities before initiating such a program within your lab.

Assuming that your state doesn't prohibit such practices, let's take a look at a case illustration to see what results you might expect to gain from such a program.

CASE IN POINT: VET TESTING PROGRAM SAVES RURAL HOSPITAL'S PATHOLOGY AND LAB PROGRAMS.

For one small midwestern hospital, the ever-increasing costs of maintaining a pathology program were becoming prohibitive. Staff salary and laboratory supply costs were creating a cost squeeze that was causing a deluge of red ink on the books of the department.

After checking regulations, this hospital initiated an innovative program to offer its lab services to veterinarians within the surrounding county, charging them a fee on the per-test basis.

Because the area had no established laboratory program for testing animal specimens, the local vets involved were very enthusiastic. Beginning with the standard pet diagnostic procedures, the hospital gradually expanded its services to include a variety of testing for horses, dairy, beef, and other animals. The program grew at a remarkable rate, due partly to the high concentration of dairy farmers in the region who needed these services.

Thanks to the foresight of this hospital administrator, the added revenue from this program (exceeding $250,000 annually) helped to put the hospital's lab on a profitable standing, canceling any plans for its elimination.

Again, one rather simple idea became the cornerstone for a major turnaround in a hospital. Using techniques which others might have rejected as unworkable, this hospital saved a vital program that would have otherwise been doomed to extinction.

Other Assorted Ideas

The utilization ideas just presented are merely only a small portion of the potential ideas which could prove to be a major factor in the financial health of your hospital. The theoretical concept of expanding any service begins with an analysis of your current levels.

You can extend these ideas to cover such diverse areas as the radiology service, accepting x-ray work from outside physicians, to the dietary department being cntracted to serve as the hot lunch source for a nearby school. The ideas which you might be able to adapt for service are virtually endless.

Suppose, for example, that you offer a day care nursery for children of hospital staff members. To cover the costs of operation, you might also wish to include children of other people within the community. By charging a small fee for this service, you can recoup the financial outlays of establishing and maintaining the program.

In addition, this could serve as an excellent public relations tool, particularly in communities that presently fail to offer such services to the public. Each time that you successfully increase the positive impact of hospital activities on the community, you will substantially benefit the efforts of fund-raising and other volunteer efforts generated by the community. This comes from the "What would we do without them?" feeling that is created within the community.

The Idea Search: Summing Up

Throughout this chapter, the emphasis has been on developing innovative new approaches to marketing the internal departmental programs of your hospital to the community outside your immediate confines. The information which we have been able to provide is merely a starting point for your deliberations on this subject.

Two essential questions are the cornerstone of any external marketing program. They are:

(1) What departmental programs within my hospital could be adapted to be useful to facilities, agencies, and individuals outside my hospital?
(2) How do I reach my targeted market effectively to deliver the message of service availability?

When you have reviewed each of your departmental services to answer these two questions, you should have a fairly accurate picture of the expansion potential which your hospital could enjoy. The revenue estimates for one hospital, due to its individuality, would not necessarily be applicable to another.

There is, however, no question as to the potential revenue expansion which all hospitals could enjoy. The only stumbling block to success in this area is a narrowness of vision, an incapacity to think in terms of "What if ...?".

If we can successfully remove the intellectual constraints which bind us to the conventional, the traditional, and the "regulation procedure," we will enjoy the blossoming of administrative innovation that makes ultimate success in an increasingly competitive health care delivery market a virtual certainty.

Adaptability is the name of the game! If you can review your programming with this in mind, your planning effectiveness will proportionally increase, making your hospital prosper while other similar hospitals flounder in the Sea of Progress.

The challenge lies before you. Answer it firmly—and with confidence! The best is yet to come.

Physician recruitment: unveiling the secrets of success

IN THIS, OUR FINAL CHAPTER, we come to the final element which is required for successful hospital management, successful physician and specialist recruitment. No matter how great your facilities, the atmosphere for physician retention, etc., the ongoing realities of marching time, natural attrition of physicians, or fundamental changes in their plans will inevitably result in a need for new practitioners for your hospital.

Your preparation, far in advance of the doctor's departure, will ensure the smoothest possible transition from Old Guard to New for your hospital. Each time there is a noticeable change in hospital staffing, with a resulting change in thinking and ideals, a hospital goes through a metamorphosis—a sort of evolutionary process—which will determine the future course of hospital policy. Your ability to analyze these impending changes, before they happen, can determine whether the future controls you, or the other way around.

At the time that this was being written, there existed a marked shortage of competently trained practitioners to fill available hospital openings in the United States. This has resulted in considerable competition for new medical school graduates, the most intense recruiting pressure coming from non-urban hospitals which face the greatest recruiting difficulties.

While the current picture for recruitment is not particularly bright, the prognosis for the future could be considered markedly more favorable. Current indicators point to a potential oversupply of medical school graduates ten to 20 years from now. This will mean a radical change in the methods of recruiting, in addition to the more favorable managerial relationship which each hospital administrator will enjoy with his medical and surgical staff.

This chapter will review the essential secrets of meeting the short-term problems of physician recruitment, as well as discuss the strategic changes which the potential future oversupply will create.

245

Elements of the Successful Recruitment Program

Developing a successful recruitment program for medical personnel is a multi-faceted concept which, though centered with hospital administration, works to combine the elements of community and hospital resources to create the most attractive picture of the opportunity possible. By using the combined approach between these two sectors, you can cover the essential elements which will go into any doctor's decision on where he will locate and develop his medical practice.

To develop this idea just a bit further, let's take a more detailed look at the factors which a physician or specialist will take into account when deciding to locate—or not locate—his activities in your area and, most important, at your hospital.

The Physician's Expected Daily Activities

Contrary to many prevailing ideas on the subject, the general scope of activities which the medical professional is called upon to perform is not a major determining factor in their decision to locate at a particular hospital. Usually, there is very little difference between a doctor's or specialist's activities whether he (or she) is located in a small town in Minnesota or a major metropolitan center like New York or Chicago.

Leisure time interests often have a greater impact on the ultimate decision of where to locate. For example, an interest in fishing would make a doctor inclined to locate next to, or within easy driving distance of, a lake. Another example might be an interest in skiing. This doctor would be inclined to locate in an area which has facilities to match his interests.

Because these same factors often play an important role in a student's decision on which university or medical school to attend, a hospital administrator might be well advised to attempt matching his surroundings to those of the medical school from which he attempts to recruit a new doctor or specialist.

To take a valid example, a medical student who would have an interest in winter activities would be most likely to attend a school where these would be available. By contrast, a student who prefers a year-round summer climate would tend to gravitate toward schools in the southern areas of the country. This would be your first key to matching your available resources with the interests of your prospective recruit.

A second potential source of information might prove to be the student Information Office at the university. Many colleges maintain a student personality profile file on students. These profiles are compiled through answers from student questionnaires regarding interests, goals, and other perceptions, which they express upon admission. While this source might not be the most reliable, due to changes in ideas which can occur during the educational process, they do offer some key to the general interests upon which you can play during the recruiting process.

From this base, studying your potential marketing target group, your approach should be similar to that utilized by a tourist information bureau, emphasizing the benefits of your area and your hospital. The only difference is in the objective. You want these people to visit *and stay* in your area to serve your hospital.

Obtaining Community Involvement

In developing the overall marketing strategy of your physician recruitment program, one vital link—the physician's wife and family—should never be overlooked. Because most prospective doctors who are looking for a place to set up practice are indeed married, many with one or more child, the needs of wife and family become a primary concern of the man you're recruiting.

As mentioned earlier, the scope of a doctor's daily activities does not vary to any great extent due to his location. He goes to his office and serves in the hospital to meet the physical health needs of his patients. However, for the family, there are entirely different considerations to be reckoned with. For example, the family must be concerned with the quality of schooling being offered within the area, recreational opportunities for the family among other comfort and status factors. These concerns are of primary importance to the family, which is not so deeply in work activities as the doctor.

Coordination between the administrator and other community leaders becomes very important in developing a program which shows prospective physicians' families the value of local attractions, activities, schools, and other applicable items in their daily lives. School officials, church and community leaders, and others can work together to present an attractive and effective picture of the community.

To underline the scope of this effort, let's look at one effective program to study its structure and its operations in daily practice.

CASE IN POINT: COMMUNITY RECRUITMENT BRINGS EFFECTIVE PHYSICIAN RECRUITMENT TO NORTHERN HOSPITAL.

Under the auspices of the hospital administrator in a northern rural community, an excellent local Physician Recruitment Committee was organized to combat a local doctor shortage. Tapping a source of interested community volunteers, including some community leaders and school officials, a"guided tour"-type program was organized to bring an attractive view of area merits to prospective doctors.

The program begins with an Open Home program that opens a resident's home to the visiting doctor and his family. While the doctor is in the area to study the prospects for permanent location, he and his family stay at this volunteer home.

The resident volunteers assist the doctor in transportation to the hospital and local facilities where he might wish to set up his office. These services are all done completely free of charge to the hospital or the doctor.

While the doctor is studying his prospects, the volunteer family is working to "sell" the doctor's family on the merits of the school system and other facets of community life. Meetings with local school officials, plus tours of the facilities, are arranged to permit the wife and children to assess the nature and extent of available opportunities for education.

The combined efforts and hospitality of the community volunteers and the hospital staff have proven beneficial. From a serious shortfall in physician staffing, this committee, in a period of a few years, has more than doubled the number of doctors serving the hospital and the community.

Funding for this recruitment effort has been generated through additional volunteer efforts, the highlight of the effort being an annual musical show sponsored by the committee at the local high school auditorium. The proceeds of the event go to continue the vital work of the committee.

The concept of community involvement in the recruitment effort is vital to its success. By thus extending an extra measure of hospitality to the new doctors, the community makes them and their families feel welcome. The extra effort also creates a feeling of "indebtedness" in the visitors. They will feel that, "How can we turn down nice people like these? Let's settle here".

Community acceptance is one psychological element that all of us consider important. Getting along well with the neighbors is one major objective of any new resident. When the community makes an extra effort to make doctors and their families feel at home, this major source of concern becomes a minor one. Often the location which makes the family happiest is the one chosen by the doctor.

Facility Modification

Though basic structural specification for most of the major medical functions of the hospital do not vary from one location to another, available equipment is usually the more pressing consideration for incoming doctors. This is particularly true of those involved in the medical specialties.

For example, attracting a gynecologist to the hospital would require that your hospital is equipped with the special instruments commonly used in gynecological procedures. This usually does not entail major cash outlays because the basic setup for operating rooms would remain the same.

Some specialties would however require more extensive modifications if current equipment does not meet requirements. The heart specialist would be a prime example of this type of case. The complex equipment required to perform open heart procedures would entail some basic modifications in the operating room, particularly if this room is not very large. The equipment involved would require quite a bit of space.

In most cases, though, the modifications would normally be minimal. Most structures today are built to make modification as simple as possible. The usual case would involve only the purchase of sufficient equipment to meet the specific needs of the incoming doctor. Most often, these are purchased *after* the doctor makes a *firm commitment* to practice in the hospital.

Financial Inducements

One problem commonly faced by the doctor is the question of financial stability during any location change. Particularly true of doctors who are already established, this also poses some problems for those fresh out of medical school. These recruits want to be sure that their basic financial needs will be met during the crucial transition period when they are developing their future practices in the area.

While some hospital managers and controllers may express reservations about it, one increasingly popular technique for surmounting this problem is the use of *monetary guarantees*. Using this method, a hospital makes a commitment to the incoming doctor for a one to three-year period, guaranteeing that the practitioner will make a certain annual income during this contract period. The common stipulations of this agreement state that the doctor must set up practice to be open to the public and serve the hospital as patient requirements dictate. In return, the hospital will assure the practitioner the agreed annual income.

Here's how this system would work. Suppose, for example, that an incoming doctor requires an annual income of $50,000. If, during his first year, the doctor only earns $45,000 from his practice and hospital activities, the hospital would be liable for the remaining $5,000 of the agreed minimum.

This "safety net" minimum setup assures that the doctor would maintain a certain standard of living, one he is probably already accustomed to, while he is setting up his practice. In most instances, though, the amount, if any, that must be made up by the hospital during the first year or two of the doctor's stay is quite nominal.

To underscore the hospital's costs in this type of inducement program, let's take a brief review of some examples:

- Midwest rural hospital offered $45,000 per year. First year cost to the hospital: $500
- Eastern hospital offered $60,000. Cost to the hospital, first year: $1,100.
- Western hospital offered $55,000. First year cost to the hospital: $225.

These examples indicate that only a small percentage of the guarantee amount is ever required to be paid by the hospital. When quality medical personnel are brought into a community, the public's use of their services often tends to grow to match the availability. This truism tends to minimize the risks of this program and makes it more attractive to hospitals considering such a move.

Frankly, we can't endorse or disavow this program based on the evidence available. All indications point toward its use only to attract established practitioners with proven track records in other areas. The use of this method with unproven young doctors just out of medical school could represent an unacceptable level of financial risk for the hospital. If the new doctor proved totally unacceptable, due to personality, a hospital could be bound to a monumentally large cash commitment with little or no chance of a future payoff on the investment.

Clearly, this recruitment technique must be classified as a gamble for any hospital. But the payoff can prove to be considerable, particularly for the hospital that is currently having serious problems with physician recruitment and retention. This guarantee mechanism might be the key, all other factors being equal, to triggering a positive response from the doctor.

Specialties: A Distinct Challenge

With a growing trend toward specialization within the medical profession, recognizing a hospital's needs in this area can be a challenging problem. While most, if not all, physicians and surgeons are fairly competent to perform the vast majority of procedures which might be encountered in daily hospital care, increasing numbers of GP's (General Practitioners) are becoming reliant on the extended knowledge of the specialist.

Due to general lack of knowledge specifically oriented to a limited portion of the body, lack of confidence in handling certain procedures, or for whatever reason, the specialist has become a vital force within almost every hospital in the country. As either a visiting consultant or resident practitioner, the specialist adds to the quantity and precision of knowledge which is available to meet patient needs.

How do you determine whether your hospital would benefit from the presence of a visiting or on-staff specialist? Begin by consulting your medical records department. If a review of these records indicates a fairly large number of referrals to other hospitals, particularly if referrals are due to the complexity of the cases, you might begin considering the possible retention of a staff specialist. This is especially true if most, if not all, of the referred cases are of a similar nature. This would clearly indicate a staff knowledge shortage in a vital area.

Meeting the Challenge

If, after your records review process, you determine that retaining a specialist would appear advisable, your next step would be consultation with your current medical staff. Getting their viewpoint on the subject, approached from the aspect of giving them "available assistance," they will probably react positively to the suggestion.

As a word of caution, we might advise you against "rubbing their noses" in the problem. Avoiding any derogatory inferences in your presentation will prevent unnecessary resistance to your plans. They probably recognized the potential problem quite a bit earlier than you did. But personal and professional pride tends to keep them from asking for the help they might readily recognize as necessary. They don't want to admit *to you* that they might be in "over their heads."

After arriving at a consensus with your current staff on the need, recruiting the specialist for your hospital can begin. Proceeding much in the same fashion as you would in recruiting a general practitioner, you begin your search for the specialist. While national and state medical societies can often serve as excellent sources of leads, one worthwhile option to consider is to advertise, in a small way, in one of the professional journals of the medical profession. In aiming for the specialist, you might seek a journal which covers the particular specialty you're seeking.

When you've received favorable responses to your queries regarding potential applicants, and having narrowed down the field (if a larger number were attracted by your job offer), you come to the time of "hard bargaining." Applicants who respond for specialty positions are most often established professionals at their current locations. Inducing them to move to your area involves a combination of environmental, physical, and financial factors. Very few specialists would be willing to change locations at a financial sacrifice.

Here is the point where the financial "guarantee" program mentioned earlier in this chapter might make a fair amount of sense. Offering a financial guarantee to the incoming specialist would definitely make the proposed location change attractive. The guarantee program could become the cornerstone of your drive to retain the specialist for your hospital.

Recruiting Strategies: Changes in the Wind

As mentioned at the outset of this chapter, the current recruiting picture for physicians is not the best. But there is a considerable amount of hope for the future. Dramatic changes in physician supply are currently developing which could have a major effect on the number, type, and ease of availability of physicians for your hospital.

According to a September, 1980, study by the Graduate Medical Education Advisory Committee (published in the January 16, 1981, issue of *Hospitals*, the supply of physicians is expected to increase 41 percent between 1980 and 1990. The study projects a national *surplus* of 60,000 doctors by 1990. This expands to a 130,000 doctor surplus by the year 2000.

How will this affect your recruiting strategy? Experts who have analyzed this situation indicate that the projected surplus will result in a greater willingness to accept hospital staff positions, based on salary considerations. The basic rule of free enterprise, "When supply exceeds demand, the price goes down," would indicate less difficulty in maintaining cost containment on medical expenses in the future.

This does *not* mean that *every* hospital will have physician applicants "beating their doors down" to get a job. Many hospitals, particularly those further removed from metropolitan areas, may still need to aggressively recruit members for their medical staffs.

The main change will come to the new doctor's greater willingness to consider working in a smaller, possibly less glamorous, hospital. If your hospital is not nationally famous, large, or otherwise offers possible avenues to gain notice, many doctors today might not even take the time to consider your offer.

Ten years or more into the future, according to the study's statistics, we may have a growing trend to the salaried hospital physician, one who is more subject to administrative controls and less independent than is currently the rule. Provided that administrative policy does not become excessively overbearing in an attempt to capitalize on this apparent supply shift, most doctors will probably opt for maintaining longevity at one hospital, becoming less mobile.

This would mean a greater emphasis on recruiting the medical school graduates or those completing residency programs. This shift in recruiting tactics would place a premium on administrators and hospital public relations people who can build and maintain effective ties with the university setting.

Considering the projections on physician supply, an apparently smart move would be to develop these liaisons *now*, if they have not been developed already. With established links to the academic community, you can bring about a gradual change in recruiting practices that ongoing physician supply conditions would dictate.

While projections of 60,000 surplus physicians for 1990 may be a fairly accurate estimate, we would be presumptuous to plan on the 130,000 figure for the year 2000. Budgetary constraints and supply considerations in the job market may precipitate cutbacks in physician education programs in the future, potentially returning us to a shortage situation sometime down the road.

Our main objective is to plan effectively to maintain adequate staffing levels during the 1980's, with recruiting changes being gradually instituted as the "supply side economics" gradually begins to assert its influence on the health care delivery marketplace.

Rewards of Success: Some Final Thoughts

The successful implementation of an ongoing physician recruitment program is clearly an imperative for any hospital that wishes to maintain its standing, both professionally and financially, as a health care provider within its community. But the rewards are no more clearly underlined than in a nationwide review which indicates that each doctor in the United States who is affiliated with a hospital will generate (at the time of this writing) $302,000 annually, on the average, for his employer. This figure breaks down to a $261,000 for inpatient services and $41,000 for outpatient charges.

As a hospital's available inpatient services expand, their use usually increases proportionally as well. In clear financial terms, the physician remains the key to the financial health of the hospital.

The quality of personnel that you successfully recruit for the medical staff will play a large role in the financial levels which your facility attains. The quality of care received plays a major part in public acceptance of the hospital. Without this acceptance, particularly in a multi-hospital community, the health care provider is out of business.

That, in a nutshell, is the essence of hospital management. By combining top-quality management ideas with personnel and medical staff that are committed to the pursuit of professional excellence, the future of any hospital can be made and maintained secure.

Though the road ahead may contain numerous hidden obstacles which can cause temporary disruptions to the best-laid plans, diligent adherence to the basic principles of sound management practice will assure that the necessary steady course of administrative planning and policy can be maintained.

Our mutual goal is to guide you through these hazards to a smoother roadway in the future. We hope this book will assist you toward this goal.

Index

INDEX

A

Abuse:
  child, 200, 203
  spouse, 200, 203-205

Accident cases, 212
Accidents, 100
Accounting department:
  combining ideas, 75-76
  computers, 72
  "continuous" forms, 72-74
  "pacemaker," 72
  paper work, 72
  "semi-computer" technology, 74-75
  third-party payment process, 78
  time required for billing, 72
  workload, 72

Administrative area, lab, 163
Administrative functions, records,
     119-120
Administrative policy, 24
Administrator, today's, 39
Admission, authorization, 116
Admitting Office:
  computer's memory bank, 70
  first contact, 70
  friendly and sympathetic attitude, 70
  impediments, 71
  information gathering, 70
  key $ and timesaver, 71-72
  patient's ability to pay, 71
  personnel, demeanor, 71
  photocopies, 72
  policy requirements, 71
  public relations, 70
  repeating similar questions, 70
  speed and competency, 70

Admitting Office, *(cont.)*
  tension factor, 70
  trivia to minimum, 70

Ambulance arrivals, 154
Ambulance drivers and attendants, 232
Ambulance service, 224
Animals, lab, 165
"Arm twisting" method, 23
Attitude, administrator, 102, 103
Audio-visual material, 225-226
Authorization, admission, 116

B

Bacteriology, 163-164
Bake sales, 233
Basal metabolism-electrocardiography
     room, 163
Battered Wives' Shelters, 203-205
Beds, empty, 34
Benefits, 24, 54-55, 63
Billing, direct, 79-80
Billing systems, shared, 53
Bingo game, 233, 241-242
Biochemistry, 163, 164
Blood Bank, 30, 31, 163
Blue Cross, 37-38
Board-granted authority, 106
Board of trustees:
  administration, relationship, 66
  basis for selection, 57
  close scrutiny of proposals, 59
  commonly recognized bylaws, 59
  composition, 56-57
  continuing education, 58-59
  continuity vs. "new blood," 57-58
  decisions in medical matters, 57
  detailed reports, 59

Board of trustees, *(cont.)*
 endowments, 57
 executive committee, 60
 experience, 57
 favoritism and "conflict of interest,"
  63-65
 finance committee, 61-62
 formal presentation, 62-63
 formation, 56-57
 full time chief executive officer, 57
 generalized holdings, 57
 hospital investments, 57
 implementing plans, 56
 joint conference committee, 60
 lapse between terms, 58
 medical memberships, 57
 meeting administrative objectives, 56
 microcosm of social structure of
  community, 57
 mutual trust and rapport, 62
 no noticeable changeover, 58
 number of members, 56
 organizational principles, 59
 preparation of presentations, 56
 primary responsibility to community,
  56
 professional committee, 60-61
 rotate membership, 58
 segmented into smaller committees,
  59
 "sell" your proposals to board, 56
 serving in voluntary capacity, 56
 single large turnover, 57
 special interests and skills, 57
 stable management policy, 58
 streamlined legislative process, 59
 support and concurrence, 56
 ultimate authority for hospital
  policies, 56
 volunteer portion, 57

Breakage, equipment, 99
Broadcasting, educational, 241-242
Budget:
 capital outlay, 88-89
 Capital Outlay Budget, 85, 86
 communications, 85
 departmental, 82-87

Budget, *(cont.)*
 first signs of crisis, 90
 hospital resurrection, 88-89
 miscellaneous (contingency fund),
  86-87
 nursing service, 151
 projected energy expenditures, 86
 projected replacement of equipment,
  85-86
 salaries of staff, 83-84
 supplies, cost, 84-85
 total, developing, 87-88
 wrapping up process, 91

Business administration, 39
Business manager, 68
Business Office, 240-241 *(see also*
  Financial Services)
Buying plan, co-op, 54

C

Cadence adaptation, 213
Cafeteria, employee, 196
Cancer, 177
Cancer research, 118
Candy Stripers, 232
Capital outlay budget, 85, 86, 88-89
Carbon copies, 71
Cardiac care, 222
Cardiopulmonary resuscitation, 223,
  229, 230
Cassette tape recorders, 120-121
Cause of Death, 161-162
Ceiling, laundry, 140
Chain of command, 42
Changes, selling, 24
Chaplaincy, 237-238
Chief of Social Services, 201, 202
Chief of Staff:
 food preparation, 190
 medical, 42-43

Child abuse, 200, 203
Childbirth classes, 223, 229, 230
Cleaning, 132
Clinical lab, 161
Clinical pathology, 30-31, 161

Collections, 79-80
Communications:
  budget, 85
  business manager, 68
  "Closed Mind-Open Mouth"
    syndrome, 22
  Dietary Department, 28, 29
  importance, 21
  internal educational broadcasting
    system, 241
  Medical Records, 29
  medical staff, 51-52
  open lines, 22

Compassion, nursing, 160
Computers:
  accounting, 72, 74, 75, 78-79
  financing, 241
  laboratory, 170
  monitoring energy use, 129
  purchasing area, 109-111
  radiology, 175
  revolution, 121-122

Conferences, 29
Confidence, 24
Conflict of interest, 63, 64-65
Contingency Fund, 86-87
Continuity, 57
"Continuous" forms, 72
Contract services, 126-127
Contributions, soliciting, 99
Controller, 68-69
Convicts, 146, 148
Co-operative purchasing agreements,
    53-54
Coroner, 162
Cost factors, 107-108
Credentials Committee, 44-45
Credit and collections:
  chronic deadbeats, 79
  deposit system, 80
  direct billing of patient, 79
  firm financial arrangements, 80
  hospital's image, 80
  interest charge problem, 80
  nonpayment, 79-80
  prevention, 80

Credit and collections, *(cont.)*
  those having financial difficulty, 79
  uninsured amounts, 80

Criminals, 146, 148
Critically ill patients, 201
CVA (stroke), 212, 217

D

Darkroom, 174-175
*Darling vs. Charleston Community
    Hospital,* 61
Data Card, 109
Day care nursery, 243
Day Care Rehabilitation Center,
    219-220
Death, Cause of, 161-162
Departmental requirements:
  dietary department, 28-29
  emergency service, 31-32
  laboratories, 30-31
  medical library, 32
  medical records, 28, 29-30
  medical social services, 33
  optional medical services, 32-33
  outpatient, 32-33
  pharmacy, 30
  radiology, 31
  rehabilitation, 33

Departmental stereotypes, 239-240
Deposit system, 80
Diagnosis, changes, 190
Dietary Department:
  auxiliary functions, 192
  centralized dietary service, 195
  changes in diagnosis, 190
  communications, 28, 29
  conferences, 29
  contracted services, 194
  cost of inefficiency, 28-29
  dietician, 29, 189, 190-192 *(see also
    Dietician)*
  feeding hired help, 195-196
  food preparation process, 192-193
  food procurement process, 190

Dietary Department, *(cont.)*
    food service manager, 189, 192
    food storage, 192
    frozen foods, 198
    hot lunches for nearby school, 243
    implementer of planning, 189
    integrated with other departments,
        28
    inventory, 191
    jail inmate feeding program, 197-198
    kitchen equipment maintenance, 192
    labor trouble, 23
    maximum productivity, 192
    minimum requirements, 28-29
    organized system, 28
    per capita cost level, 189
    "professional" image, 193
    qualified personnel, 28
    record of diets, 29
    reputation for better wages, 193-194
    revenue-producing programs,
        196-198
    sanitation, 29, 192
    staffing levels, 192-194
    vending machines, 192
    waste, 190

Dietician:
    administrative ability, 191
    amounts of food prepared, 190
    changes in diagnosis, 190
    "Chief of Staff," 190
    communication with business office,
        190
    consulting-service, 191
    department records, 191
    designs patients' diets, 190
    food procurement, 190
    formulates hospital's menu, 189
    head of department, 189
    if none is available, 191
    inventory, 191
    part-time, 191
    Patient Census, 190
    shared-service, 191
    single position, 190
    waste, 190

Drainage, laundry, 140

Drugs, 30, 143-144 *(see also* Pharmacy)
Dying patients, 201

E

Education:
    audio-visual material, 225
    budget, 225
    cardiac care, 222
    certification training programs, 222
    childbirth classes, 223, 229
    community, 223, 229-230
    Community Tuition Grant systems,
        228
    CPR classes, 223, 229, 230
    duplication, 224
    employee retention, 223
    expanding horizons, 228-229
    external resources, 230-231
    "faculty," 224
    greater efficiency, 223
    hospital policy, 100
    individual department chiefs, 224
    in-service training, 223-225
    instruction seminars, 224
    internal broadcasting system, 241
    larger hospitals, 224
    long-range outlook, 223
    lower patient care costs, 223
    mandated requirements, 224
    medical and related, 116-117
    medical library, 228-229
    nursing, 222, 223
    ostomy classes, 223, 230
    paramedics, ambulance teams, 224
    peripheral support services, 224
    "prevention ethic," 229
    reducing literature involved, 225
    regionalized information centers, 230
    renal function, 222
    "satellite" training program, 227-228
    single directorship, 224
    smaller hospitals, 224
    total start-up investment, 225
    training films, 225
    training location, 224
    transportation of employees, 224
    videocassette system, 225, 226

Efficiency:
    housekeeping, 132-137
    laundry and linen, 137-142
    security service, 142-149

Electronic schematic diagrams, 125
Electronic typewriter, 74, 75
Emergency Entrance, 154
Emergency service, 31-32
Emotional detachment, 25
Empathy, 202
Employee:
    morale, 102
    services, 96-97
    training, 100

Employment, initial, 94-95
Empty beds, 34
Endowments, 57
Energy, expenditures, 86
Energy situation, 128-129
Engineer, 125

Engineering and maintenance:
    control mechanisms, 129-130
    detailed cost analytical material, 129
    electronic schematic diagrams, 125
    energy question, 128-129
    "Extended Warranty," 126
    files, 125-126
    graduate engineer, 125
    hidden costs, 129
    in-house, 127-128
    increased hospitalization, 129
    internal department vs. contract
        services, 126-127
    inventory listings, 129
    lost time, 129
    maintenance schedules, 125
    major equipment purchases, 125
    manuals or guides, 125
    microcomputers, 129
    most current technological
        information, 124
    night shift, 125
    one staffer per one hundred beds,
        125
    organization and staffing, 124-125
    outgoing paper work, 129

Engineering and maintenance, *(cont.)*
    parts and supply requisitions, 129
    periodic reports, 129
    plant operations supervisor, 124-125
    prevention, 125-126
    quality of care, 129
    recorded information, 125-126
    reliance on technology, 124
    savings, 127-128
    "temporary" repairs, 126
    "Time Factor," 127
    training, 124, 125
    24-hour-a-day coverage, 125
    working drawings and floor plans,
        125

Enthusiasm:
    can turn the tide, 25
    marks successful people, 25
    project, 21

Equipment:
    breakage, 99
    incoming doctors, 248
    projected replacement, 85-86

Evacuation, fire, 135, 143, 144, 145-146
Executive Committee, 43, 60
Experience, 57, 92
Extended Care, 34-35
"Extended Warranty," 126

F

Favoritism, 63-64
Federal health care, 34
Felons, 146
Films, training, 225, 226
Finance Committee, 61
Financial inducements, physicians,
    248-249
Financial Services:
    accounting department, 72-76
        combining ideas, 75-76
        "continuous" forms, 72-74
        "semi-computer" technology, 74-75
    Admitting Office, 70-72
    business manager, 68
    controller, 68-69

Financial Services, *(cont.)*
  C.P.A., 68
  credit and collections, 79-80
  functions within office, 69-81
  key $ and timesaver, 71-72
  leadership, 68
  other functions, 80-81
  paper traffic center, 76
  payroll function, 76-78
  primary functions, 67-68
  third-party payment process, 78-79
  you and controller, 69

Fire safety:
  ambulatory patients, 135
  bed patients, 135
  central fire panel, 144-145
  evacuation, 135, 143, 144, 145-146
  flammable substances, 135
  housekeeping's duties, 135
  meetings, 145, 146
  patients requiring oxygen, 146
  planning, 145-146
  police or security personnel, 143,
          144, 145-146
  regulations, 146
  State Fire Marshall, 146

Floor plans, 125
Floors, laundry, 140
Fluid Science, 161
Food *(see* Dietary Department)
Frozen foods, 198
Fund-raising, 232, 233

G

General Practitioners, 250
Germ control, 132
Gift Shop, 233
Glasswashing, 164-165
Goals:
  myth of "Overnight Success," 24
  realistic, 24-25
  short-and long-range, 25
  time allotted for attainment, 25

Government intervention, 34

Gratuities, 99

Group buying:
  effective alternative, 111-112
  legal obligations, 112-113
  management consortium, 112

Guarantees, 108
Guides, equipment, 125
Gynecology services, 154

H

Handbook for Hospital Trustees, 59
Handwriting, illegible, 120-121
Head nurse, 152
Health, 97
Health care plans, 21, 34, 36-38
Health is a Community Affair, 58
Health Maintenance Organization,
        37-38
Heart surgery, 117
Hematology, 163
Holdings, 57
Holidays, 97
Home care, 203
Hospital Guild, 232, 233-234
Hospitalization, 97
Hospital Policy Decisions—Process and
        Action, 59
Hospital Trusteeship, 59
Hours, working, 98
Housekeeping:
  cleaning rags, 136
  fire and safety duties, 135
  flammable substances, 135
  friendly competition, 134
  general cleaning, 132
  germ control, 132
  Head Housekeeper, 133
  incentives, 134
  individual pride, 134
  infection control, 132
  Linen and Laundry section, 136,
        137-142 *(see also* Laundry
        and Linen)
  productivity, better, 134

Housekeeping, *(cont.)*
   role in evacuation, 135
   room preparation, 132
   sewing room, 136
   structure, staff, 132-133
   team concept, 134-135
   training, staff, 133-134
   waste, slashing, 134

Human Resources Director, 92-93 *(see
   also* Personnel)

I

Ideas:
   benefits, 24
   counterproductive, 25
   encourage, 22

Image, self-, 22
Incentive programs, 23, 134
Infection Committee, 48-49
Infection control, 132
Influenza, 132
Information centers, 230-231
Information gathering, 70
Injuries, 99-100
In-service training, 223-225
Inspection, merchandise, 108
Insurance:
   liability, 177
   public, 167-168

Insurance programs, 36-37
Intensive Care Program for Relatives,
   201
Intensive Care Unit, 152, 153
Interest charge, 80
Internship program, nurse, 157-158
Inventory *(see* Purchasing)
Investments, 57
Involvement, active, 52

J

Jail inmate feeding program, 197
Job analysis and description, 101
Joint Conference Committee, 44, 60

L

Laboratories, 30-31
Laboratory services:
   administrative, 163
   animals, 165
   Bacteriology, 163, 164
   basal metabolism-
        electrocardiography room,
        163
   Biochemistry, 163, 164
   Blood Bank, 163
   Cause of Death, 161-162
   clinical lab, definition, 161
   clinical pathology, definition, 161
   computer, 170
   Coroner or Medical Examiner, 162
   cost controls, 169-170
   departmental organization, 162
   dynamics of expanded service,
       165-166
   expansion of floor plan, 162
   Fluid Science, 161
   forms and records, 168-169
   glasswashing and sterilization,
       164-165
   Hematology, 163
   innovations, 242-243
   laboratory assistants, 162
   Medicaid, 167
   medical technologists, 162
   Medicare, 167
   morgue, 165
   necroscopy, 165
   Parasitology, 163
   pathologist, 162
   pathologist's office, 163
   public health reimbursement system,
       167
   public insurance and laboratory
       crisis, 167-168
   Serology, 163, 164
   specimen storage, 165
   specimen toilet, 163
   technical area, 163-164
   Unitized Design Concept, 163-164
   variable layout planning, 162-165

Laboratory services, *(cont.)*
   venipuncture cubicle, 163
   vet testing programs, 242-243
   waiting room, 163

Labor policies, 97
Labor trouble, 23
"Last hired—first fired" ethic, 94
Laundry and Linen:
   "check in and out" system, 139
   commercial laundry, 139
   computerization, 139
   consolidated laundry services,
         139-140, 141-142
   cost, 138-139, 142
   daily laundry load, 138
   damaged linen, 139
   distribution, 137
   drainage, 140
   employee: bed ratio, 138
   floors, 140
   housekeeping, 136
   internal features of laundry, 140
   lighting, 141
   locating in-hospital laundry, 140
   manager, 137
   moisture-resistant materials, 140
   monitoring quality, 139
   obstetrics activity, 138
   organization and staffing, 137-139
   output, improving, 141
   Patient Census, 138
   sample laundry plan, 138
   sheets, 137
   slack times, 141
   slatted wood platforms, 141
   small hospital, 139
   sufficient supplies, 137
   surgical activity, 138
   trade association, 137
   trade journals, 137
   uniforms, 137
   wall and ceiling materials, 140
   windows, 141

Law enforcement, 203
Leadership, financial services, 68
Leave, sick, 98

Leave of absence, 98-99
Legal considerations, records, 118-119
Library, medical, 228-229
Licensed Practical Nurses, 152
Lighting, laundry, 141
Limb, loss, 212
Linen *(see* Laundry and Linen)

M

Maintenance and engineering, 124-130
      (see also Engineering and
      maintenance)
Malpractice claims, 118
Management:
   advancements, 21
   incentive programs, 23
   medical core, 40-55 *(see also* Medical
      staff)
   objectives, 92-93

Manuals:
   equipment, 125
   nursing, 158-160

Materials management *(see* Purchasing)
Medicaid, 34, 39, 167
Medical administration, 39
Medical Audit Committee, 47-48
Medical Examiner, 162
Medical library, 32
Medical Records Administrator:
   administrative functions, 119-120
   center of action, 114-115
   computers, 121-122
      automatic filing, 121
      cost effectiveness, 121-122
      high prime lending rate, 122
      larger hospitals, 122
      micro-circuitry, 121
      physical size, 121
      proliferation of companies, 122
      reduced storage space, 121
      speed of information retrieval, 121
   departmental operating objectives,
      115-120
   doctors dictate onto cassette, 120-121

Medical Records Administrator, *(cont.)*
  illegible handwriting, 120-121
  legal considerations, 118-119
  Library Science, 115
  Medical Terminology, 115
  Management Objectives, 115
  medical and related education,
    116-117
  multi-purposes of hospital records,
    116
  patient care, 115-116
  problem solving, 122-123
  research, 117-118

Medical Records Committee, 45-47
Medical Records Department:
  central purpose, 29
  communications, 29
  identification system for all records,
    29
  indexing method, 29
  interconnection point for dietary
    department, 28
  minimum requirements, 29-30
  nomenclature, 29
  operational flow pattern, 29
  organization, 29
  peak performance, 30
  relationship with medical and/or
    surgical staff, 29-30
  speedy retrieval of record, 29
  staffing, 29

Medical section, rehabilitation, 212
Medical services, 34
Medical Social Services Department, 33
Medical staff:
  benefits, 54-55
  Chief of Staff, 42-43
  co-operative purchasing agreement,
    53-54
  Credentials Committee, 44-45
  executive committee, 43
  getting actively involved, 52
  improved communication, 51-52
  individual needs of hospital, 51
  Infection Committee, 48-49
  internal organization, 42

Medical staff, *(cont.)*
  Joint Conference Committee, 44
  Medical Audit Committee, 47-48
  Medical Records Committee, 45-47
  organizing, 41-51
  "politics" and medical standards, 41
  potential for friction, 51
  responsibility, 41
  shared billing systems, 53
  social services, 202-203
  strengthen ties to hospital, 52-54
  Tissue Committee, 47
  Utilization Committee, 49-50
  working relationship with, 51-55

Medical technologists, 162
Medicare, 34, 36, 37, 39, 167
Medications, 30, 143-144 *(see also*
    Pharmacy)
Mediocrity, 25
Merit rating system, 96
Miscellaneous, budget, 86-87
Monetary guarantees, 249
Money, employee relations, 22-24
Morale, employee, 102
Morgue, 165
Motivation:
  "arm twisting," 23
  before making presentation, 24
  communication, 21, 22
  confidence projects itself, 24
  confident command of facts, 24
  cost control angle, 23
  employees monitor each other, 22
  enthusiasm, 21, 25
  failure, 22
  goals, 24-25
    "Overnight Success," 24
    realistic, 24-25
    short- and long-range, 25
    time allotted, 25
  incentive programs, 23
  increased productivity, 21, 22, 23
  key element to success, 25
  monetary rewards, 22-24
  people with ideas, 22
  pride in job well done, 22

Motivation, *(cont.)*
  protect advancements, 21
  self-image of employee, 22
  "selling benefits," 24
  shared savings plan, 23
  total department performance, 22
  uncertainties, 24
  unionized hospital, 23

Motor-Impulse propelled prosthetics, 212
Muscle re-education, 212

N

Necroscopy, 165
Nomenclature, 29
Nursery, day care, 243
Nurses' station, 152, 153, 154, 155
Nursing, rehabilitation, 216
Nursing staff:
  adequate levels, 150, 151
  ambulance arrivals, 154
  assistant nursing director, 151
  budget, 151
  centralized facilities, 150
  central location of facilities, 152-154
  compassion, 160
  evaluation of care, 151
  head nurse, 152
  individual nurses, 152
  innovative nurse retention programs, 155-158
    nurse internship program, 157-158
    staff-initiated nursing programs, 156-157
  Intensive Care Unit, 152
  Licensed Practical Nurse, 152
  maintaining supply connection, 154-155
  morale, 154
  nurses' station, 152, 153, 154, 155
  nursing director, 150-151
  organization, 151
  patient-call monitor switchboard, 152
  patient record charts, 152
  policies, 151

Nursing staff, *(cont.)*
  procedural manuals, 158-160
  procedures, 151
  records, 151
  Registered Nurses, 152
  specialized nursing requirements, 150
  staffing levels, 155
  supervisor, 152
  supplies and equipment, 151
  unit authority substructure, 151-152
  working relationships, 151

O

Objectives, management, 92, 93
Obsolescence, 107, 108
Obstetrics services, 154
Occupancy rate, 90
Occupational Therapy, 213
Older patients, 201, 206
Organ donor programs, 201
Organization, medical staff, 41-51 *(see also* Medical staff)

Organizational structure:
  background of administrator, 39
  Dietary Department, 28-29
  emergency service, 31-32
  finding balance, 35-36
  importance, 27
  individual units, 27
  insurance programs, 36-37
  interrelationships between departments, 27
  keeping staff, 38
  laboratories, 30-31
  medical library, 32
  Medical Records Department, 28, 29-30
  minimum departmental requirements, 27-39
  optional medical services, 32-33
    Medical Social Services Department, 33
    outpatient department, 32-33
    rehabilitation department, 33

Organizational structure, *(cont.)*
  pharmacy, 30
  prepayment plans, 37-38
  problems, 27, 34-35
  radiology, 31
  service diversification, 38

Ostomy care classes, 223, 230
Outpatient, rehabilitation, 219
Outpatient Department, 32-33
Overstaffing, 90
Oxygen, patients requiring, 146

P

Packages, 99
Paper traffic center, 76
Paper work, 34
Paramedics, 224
Parasitology, 163
Pathological Anatomy, 30, 31
Pathologist, 162, 163
Patient-call monitor switchboard, 152
Patient care, 115-116
Patient Census, 90
Patient record charts, 152
Payroll function, 76-78
Peak period workloads, 239
Pediatrics rooms, 154
Peer review process, 207-208
Performance:
  minimum departmental, 27-39
  wage benefits, 23

Personnel:
  administrative role, 103
  conditions for initial employment,
      94-95
  director, 92-93
    diplomacy, 93
    judge of people and character, 93
    management objectives, 92, 93
    motivator of people, 93
    qualities and qualifications, 92-93
    recruiting function, 93
    supervisory experience, 92-93
  employee services, 96-97

Personnel, *(cont.)*
  employee training, 100
  equipment breakage, 99
  financial services, 67
  general labor policies, 97
  health and hospitalization, 97
  holidays, 97-98
  job analysis and description, 101
  "last hired-first fired" ethic, 94
  leave of absence, 98-99
  merit rating system, 96
  morale, 102-103
  policies, 93-101
  problems, 103
  prohibition of gratuities to
      employees, 99
  promotions and transfers, 95
  protection for employees' property,
      99
  safety conditions, 99-100
  salary and wages, 100-101
  sick leave restrictions and benefits, 98
  smoking restrictions, 99
  soliciting of contributions, 99
  taking packages from building, 99
  termination of employment, 95-96
  vacations, 100
  working hours, 98

Pharmacy:
  accounting, 182
  additional staffing, 185
  administrative paraphernalia, 184
  administrative reports, 187
  alarm systems, 185
  alcohol control, 182
  annual recounting of pharmacy
      activities, 187
  antidotes, 182
  assistants, 185
  authority structure, 181-182
  bed capacity, 180
  centralized location, 185
  control forms, 187
  controlled substances, 184
  dispensing drugs, 182
  drug monitoring system, 183

Pharmacy, *(cont.)*
  duplication of drugs, 182
  emergency medications, 182
  equipment installation, 185
  facilities, 183-184
  facilities maintenance, 182
  filing equipment, 184
  filling and labeling containers, 182
  furnishing pharmaceutical
          information, 182
  "generic" drugs, 185-186
    heated controversy, 185
    lower cost, 186
    standards and regulations, 185-186
    transition process, 186
    "wean" the medical staff, 186
  hospitals sharing pharmacist, 185
  in-house vs. consulting service,
          180-181
  injectable substances, 182
  inspection of pharmaceuticals, 182
  internal stock requisition, 187
  inventory listings, 187
  medications permitted, 182
  narcotics control, 182
  one staff member per 50 beds, 185
  organization, 30
  organizer, 182
  paper work, 187
  patient deaths, 183
  pharmacist's role, 182-183
  Pharmacy and Therapeutics
          Committee, 182, 183
  policy, 182, 183
  primary space consumers, 184
  record-keeping supplies, 184
  records, 182
  reports on pharmacy activities, 183
  retail pharmaceuticals merchant, 180
  security, 184-185
  semi-autonomous department, 182
  slack periods, 185
  smallest hospitals, 180, 185
  special narcotics order forms, 187
  specifications, 182
  standard pharmaceutical order

Pharmacy, *(cont.)*
      forms, 187
    state and federal regulations, 183
    storage facility walls, 185
    teaching courses, 182
    workload, 183-184

Photocopies, 72
Physical therapy, 212-213
Physician recruitment, 245-252
Plant Operations Supervisor, 124
Pneumococcal viruses, 133
Police, sharing facilities, 143, 147-149
      (see also Security)
Police agencies, rape victim, 205
Policies:
  contrasting, 65
  personnel, 93-101

Politics, staff, 41-42
Prepayment plan, 37-38
Presentation:
  before making, 24
  budget process, 91
  formal board, 62-63

Pre-vocational evaluation, 215-216
Priority system, scheduling, 218
Prison riots, 148
Problem solving, medical records,
      122-123
Procurement function, 104
Productivity, increased, 21, 22, 23, 134
Professional Committee, 60-61
Promotions, 95
Proof, records, 118
Prosthetics, 212
Psychological services, 213-214
Public health reimbursement system,
      167

Public relations:
  Admitting Office, 70
  day care nursery, 243
  sympathetic care for patient, 207

Purchasing:
  actual cost, 107

Purchasing, *(cont.)*
   board-granted authority, 106
   centralization, 105
   checking supplies carefully, 109
   computers, 109-111
   continuous inventory system, 109
   cost factors, 107-108
   Data Card, 109
   departmental requisitions, 108
   emergency requisitions, 109
   group buying, 111-113
      effective alternative, 111-112
      legal obligations, 112-113
      management corsortium, 112
   guarantees, 108
   individual department heads, 105
   initial inventory, 108
   instructions as to use of supplies, 109
   inventory control, 110-111
   items currently on inventory, 109
   items not in stock, 109
   merchandise inspection, 108
   obsolescence, 107, 108
   ongoing inventory process, 108
   outside repair services, 108
   patronage refunds, 108
   purchase order, 109
   quality, monitoring, 108
   quantity decisions, 107
   receiving report, 109
   record-keeping, 108
   responsibility, 104
   shipments to departments, 109
   "short cut" method to ordering,
      109-110
   specialized, 105
   stock record cards, 109
   stock records, 109
   storage costs, 108
   store requisition, 109
   supply management regulations,
      108-109
   supply shipments received, 109
   time using the item, 108
   transportation charges, 108
   vendor selection, 106-107

Purchasing, *(cont.)*
   weekly stockroom requisition, 109
   when requisitions arrive, 109
   work hours, receiving, 108

Purchasing agreements, 53-54

Q

Quality, supplies, 107, 108

R

Radiology:
   activities, 31
   computers, 175
   darkroom, 174-175
   departmental organization, 171-172
   facilities, 172-175
   liability insurance, 177
   office, 173
   radiographic room, 173-174
   safety cuts cost, 177
   standard policies, 176-177
   trends, 177
   viewing room, 173
   waiting room, 173
   x-ray work from outside, 243

Radio-thon, 235-236
Raffles, 233
Rape, 203, 205-206
Rapport, 62
Record charts, 152
Records:
   laboratory, 168-169
   medical, 28, 29-30 *(see also* Medical
      Records Administrator;
      Medical Records
      Department)
   nursing, 151

Recruitment:
   benefits of area and hospital, 247
   elements of successful program, 246
   facility modification, 248
   financial inducements, 248-249
   leisure time interests, 246
   local attractions, 247

Recruitment, *(cont.)*
  medical school graduates, 251
  meeting challenge, 250-251
  obtaining community involvement,
        247-248
  personality profiles, 246
  personnel director, 93
  physician, 245-252
  physician's expected daily activities,
        246-247
  recreational opportunities, 247
  salaried hospital physician, 251
  schools within area, 247
  specialties, 250
  strategies, changes, 251-252
  supply to increase, 251
  surroundings, 246
  those completing residency
        programs, 251
  wife and family of physician, 247

Refunds, patronage, 108
Regional rehabilitation center, 217-218
Registered Nurses, 152
Rehabilitation Department, 33
Rehabilitation nursing, 216
Rehabilitation services:
  costs, 219-220
  Day Care Rehabilitation Center,
        219-220
  medical section, 212
  nursing, 216
  occupational therapy, 213
  outpatient, 219
  physical therapy, 212-213
  pre-vocational evaluation, 215-216
  psychological, 213-214
  regional center concept, 217-218
  scheduling, 218-219
  short-period rehabilitation and
        therapy session, 219
  social, 214
  speech therapy, 213
  vocational counseling, 214-215
  working as total team, 216-217

Relatives, emotional support, 206
Religious holidays, 98

Renal function nursing, 222
Repairs, temporary, 126
Repair services, 108
Replacement, equipment, 85-86
Requisitions *(see* Purchasing)
Research, 117-118
Retrieval, records, 29
Revenue base:
  business office, 240-241
  dealing in specifics, 240-243
  drop departmental stereotypes,
        239-240
  hospital communications, 241-242
  laboratory innovations, 242-243
  selling the service, 240
  vet testing program, 242-243

Revenue collections, 82, 90
Rewards, monetary, 22-24

S

Safety conditions, 99-100
Salaries, staff, 83-84, 100-101
Saving plan, 23
Scheduling, rehabilitation, 218-219
Security:
  central fire panel, 144
  Chief of Security, 144
  convict crisis, 146, 148
  designated hospital zones, 144
  disaster planning, 143
  fire safety planning, 143, 144,
        145-146 *(see also* Fire safety)
  hiring security personnel, 143
  hospital-sponsored, 143-144
  illegal drug activity, 143-144
  location of office, 144
  organizing department, 144-145
  pocket pagers, 144
  rate of staffing, 144
  reassessment of policies, 142
  share facilities with police, 143,
        147-149
    attitudes, 147
    benefits, 143
    financial outlook, 143, 147

Security, *(cont.)*
    share facilities with police *(cont.)*
        response time cut, 143
        staff-police relationship, 143,
            148-149
    video cameras, 149

Self-image, 22
"Semi-computer" technology, 74
Senior citizens, 34
Seniority, 23
Serology, 163, 164
Service diversification, 38
Sewing room, 136
Shared billing systems, 53
Shared saving plan, 23
Sheets, 137
Sick leave, 98
Smoking restrictions, 99

Social services:
    adequate home care, 203
    age demographics, 201
    alliances with counseling groups, 203
    alternative care facilities, 202
    Battered Wives Shelters, 203-205
    budget, 209
    Chief of Social Services, 201, 202
    child or spouse abuse, 200, 203-205
    connections with outside, 203-205
    empathy with people, 202
    financial risks to facility, 200
    flexibility, 200
    hospital's management objectives,
        202
    hospital standards, 200
    hospital vs. community social worker,
        208-209
    law enforcement, 203
    measures of success, 200
    measuring results, 207-208
    medical, 33
    medical staff connection, 202-203
    medical staff meetings, 202
    older patients, 201, 206
    one staffer per 100-bed capacity
        ratio, 201

Social services, *(cont.)*
    organizing, 201-202
    patient's health, 202
    peer review, 207-208
    "People Connection," 209
    pressure, 202
    problem, 200
    public relations "front," 202
    "quality control," 207
    rape victim, 203, 205-206
        examination process, 205
        listening and support, 205
        no ironclad procedural rules,
            205-206
        outside agencies, 203
        pertinent information, 205
        referred, 205
    rehabilitation process, 214
    relation to outside agencies, 200
    size and organization, 201
    subordinate staff members, 202
    sympathetic attitude, 200
    terminally ill, 206-207
        emotional support for relatives,
            206-207
        public relations, 207
        tissue donor program, 206
    total health care mission, 200
    Utilization Committee, 202

Soliciting of contributions, 99
Space, 34
Specialist, recruitment, 250
Specimen storage, 165
Specimen toilet, 163
Speech therapy, 213
Spouse abuse, 200, 203
Stability of hospital, 24
Staffing levels, 90
Standards, medical, 41-42
Staphylococcus, 132
State health care, 34
Stereotypes, 239-240
Sterilization, lab, 164-165
Stock record cards, 109
Storage costs, 108
Store requisition, 109

Stroke, 212, 213
Supervisory experience, 92
Strike, 23
Supplies, cost, 84-85
Surgical services, 34

T

Tape recorders, 120-121
Team management concept, 62
"Team Unity" in employees, 134
Technical area, lab, 163-164
Television, 241
Tenure, 57
Terminally ill, 206
Tissue donor program, 206
Termination of employment, 95-96
Thefts, 147
Therapy, 213
Third-party payers, 78
Tissue Committee, 47
Today's Hospital, 58
Tongue guidance, 213
Training, 100, 125, 133-134, 222-231
     (*see also* Education)
Transfers, 95
Transition, 57
Transportation charges, 108
Trust, 62
Trustee, 59
Typewriters, 74-75

U

Uniforms, 137
Unionized employees, 23
Unitized Design Concept, 163-164

Utilization Committee, 49-50, 202
Utilization practices, 34

V

Vacations, 100
Velvet Boot Theory, 21, 92
Vendor selection, 106-107
Venipuncture cubicle, 163
Vet Testing programs, 242-243
Video cameras, 149
Videocassette system, 225, 226
Video Display Terminal, 74
Vocational counseling, 214-215
Volunteer services:
    chaplaincy, 237-238
    coordinating activities, 236
    Hospital Guild, 232, 233-234
    motivational keys, 234-236
    public relations, 243
    Radio-thon, 235
    recruiting, 234

W

Walkouts, 23-24
Walls, laundry, 140
Warranty, 126
Wildcat strike, 23
Windows, laundry, 141
Wives, battered, 203-205
Working hours, 98
Workmen's Compensation Laws, 99

X

X-ray work (*see* Radiology)